Modern world issues

Series editor: John Turner

KV-577-965

Health issues

GRAHAM PIKE

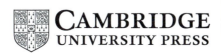
CAMBRIDGE
UNIVERSITY PRESS

071478

For Kate

Published by the Press Syndicate of the University of Cambridge
The Pitt Building, Trumpington Street, Cambridge CB2 1RP
40 West 20th Street, New York, NY 10011-4211, USA
10 Stamford Road, Oakleigh, Melbourne 3166, Australia

© Cambridge University Press 1994

First published 1994

Printed in Great Britain by Scotprint Ltd, Musselburgh

A catalogue record for this book is available from the British Library

Library of Congress cataloging in publication data applied for

ISBN 0 521 40869 5 paperback

Acknowledgements

Photographs: 9*t*, Unicef/Arild Vollan/8720; 9*b*, Unicef/Sean Sprague (82)/8943; 11*b*, Andrew Watson/Life File; 17, Unicef/Bernard Wolf/6027; 21, Unicef/Margaret Olah; 26, Miguel Arana/Life File; 27, Mary Evans Picture Library; 29, Piers Cavendish/Impact Photos; 36*t*, Colorsport/© Duomo; 36*b*, 54, Steve Benbow/Impact Photos; 42, Unicef/David Mangurian/6651; 44, Mark Edwards/Still Pictures; 52, Mike Evans/Life File; 53, Unicef/Maggie Black/242-83; 55, Joanne O'Brien/Format; 57, Unicef/Bernard P. Wolff (81)/8748; 60, Unicef/Osei G. Kofi/4158-36A; 64*r*, Unicef/Shamsuz Zaman/3308-90; 64*l*, Unicef; 65, Unicef/Carolyn Watson/3181-89.

Illustrations: 11*t*, Borgman, reproduced in *Thin Black Lines*, Development Education Centre, Birmingham; 13, *New Internationalist*, November 1986; 16*t*, Unicef/Unep, 1990; 16*b*, *New Internationalist*, November 1991; 19, *The State of the World's Children 1991*, Unicef/OUP; 25, reproduced with permission from the Health Education Authority; 28, *Tobacco Reporter*, January 1990; 30*t*, Ken Pyne; 30*b*, *World Health Forum*, WHO, Vol. 9, 1988; 34, *The Independent*, October 1991; 38, Ministry of Health, Nairobi; 43*t*, *New Internationalist*, May 1990; 48, *Witch Doctor?*, Century, 1985; 49, Mr Cecil Rajendra, first published in *Bones & Feathers* HEB (Asia) Ltd in 1978; 50, Brooks, reproduced in *Thin Black Lines*, Development Education Centre, Birmingham; 51, Oliphant, reproduced in *Thin Black Lines*, Development Education Centre, Birmingham; 56, Boy Dominuez, *Health Alert*; 59, Hesperian Foundation; 61, Pluto Press, 1986; 62, Hesperian Foundation; 63, *New Internationalist*, January 1992; 65*b*, Laxman, reproduced in *Thin Black Lines*, Development Education Centre, Birmingham; 68, 71, Random House; 72, WHO Regional Office for Europe, Copenhagen.

Cover: scanner: Mike Evans/Life File; primary health care: Unicef/Alastair Matheson/5762-5770

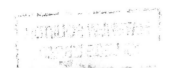

Contents

Part one   Health and ill-health

1 Health care around the world 5
What is health? 5
The state of the world's health 6
Healthy, wealthy and wise? 8
Basic needs 9
External pressures 10
Choices 12

2 Disease and disability 13
The causes of disease 13
The diseases of poverty 15
The diseases of affluence 18
Mental illness and disability 20
Priorities in the 1990s 22

Part two   Major health issues

3 Smoking: a preventable epidemic? 24
Cigarettes – legal but deadly 24
The fashionable drug 26
Tobacco is big business 27
The politics of smoking 29

**4 AIDS: world health's greatest
    challenge** 31
The short history of AIDS 31
Devastating consequences 33
The 20th-century plague 35
Fighting ignorance: condoms and cassava
    leaves 36
Chasing a cure: the big divide 39

5 The environmental connection 40
Environment . . . the key to health 40

Water – a matter of life and death 41
Air – a chemical cocktail 44
Toxic waste – the price of progress? 47

6 The People versus HealthCare plc 50
The economic argument 50
The technological argument 52
The moral argument 54
The commercial argument 55

Part three   New directions in health care

**7 Primary health care: putting people
    first** 58
Community health workers 59
Focus on women 61
Education: essential for health 62
Progress in primary health care 64

**8 Alternative medicine: treating whole
    people** 66
Traditional medicine 66
Alternative medicine 68
Naturopathy: helping yourself to good
    health 70
Complementary medicine: the best of both
    worlds? 70

9 Health for all in the 21st century 72
The story so far 72
Healthy person, healthy planet 73
Towards the 'Healthy School' 75

Further resources on health issues 77

Index 80

Health is . . .

LOOKING GOOD

FEELING 100% FIT

Eating the right food

BEING VALUED

Having adequate food, water and clothing

A BALANCE BETWEEN WORK AND PLAY

Not abusing your body

A state of complete physical, mental and social well-being (W.H.O.)

ABSENCE OF DISEASE

1   Health care around the world

What is health?

'You'll ruin your health!'
'At least I've got my health.'
'Are you in good health?'

What is meant by the word 'health' in these common phrases and sayings? Whereas we might all agree that our health is important to us, there would probably be some disagreement about what we mean exactly by 'health'. The state of our health preoccupies each of us daily, from attention to personal hygiene, fitness and diet to consumption of medicines, pills and lotions. We are bombarded with advice – some of it contradictory – from teachers, parents, friends and doctors. Advertisements attempt to lure us into buying certain products with the assurance that they will make us feel better, or look better, or smell nicer. We are told, too, about the 'risks' to our health, from smoking, alcohol and drugs; from not eating well or not sleeping enough; from inadequate exercise or too much stress. It might well be assumed, from the amount of time, effort and money spent on it, that each of us has a clear idea of what health is and how to achieve or maintain it. But just as 'beauty is in the eye of the beholder', so 'health' is open to just as many interpretations.

For the majority of the world's people, health is not a question of looking or feeling better but a matter of basic survival. In countries and communities where there is insufficient food, where water is contaminated and disease is an everyday fact of life, the pursuit of health takes on a different meaning altogether. Nonetheless, it is useful to have a definition of health which is generally accepted throughout the world. The World Health Organisation (WHO), the United Nations body founded in 1948 to help realise 'the attainment by all peoples of the highest possible level of health', defines health as 'a state of complete physical, mental and social well-being'. It recognises, however, that different countries will achieve different levels of health according to their prevailing social, economic and environmental circumstances. The Thirtieth World Health Assembly in 1977 decided to set a more specific target for WHO and for governments, namely 'the attainment by all citizens of the world by the year 2000 of a level of health that will permit them to lead a socially and economically productive life'. This goal, which has become known as 'health for all by the year 2000', has shaped and inspired the health policies and strategies of many nations for more than a decade. As the year 2000 approaches, this book assesses the worldwide progress made towards the achievement of that goal.

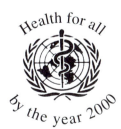

5

The *developing world* includes all the poorer countries of Africa, Asia and Latin America. It is often called the *Third World*. The very poorest parts of the developing world – predominantly in Africa – are referred to as the *least developed countries*. The *industrialised countries* are the wealthy nations of Europe, North America, Australasia and Japan. These categories are only useful in general terms, as there are many anomalies. The oil-rich countries of the Middle East are among the wealthiest on earth but in other respects they are similar to poorer nations. We should remember too that there are rich and poor people in most nations. Other terms used in this book are *the North* or *the rich world* for the industrialised countries and *the South* or *the poor world* for the developing nations.

This map clearly shows the division between the industrialised countries ('the North') and the developing countries ('the South'). The map, based on the Peters projection, has distorted the shape of the countries but gives an accurate picture of their surface area.

The state of the world's health

Is it totally unrealistic to expect ever to reach the goal of 'complete physical, mental and social well-being' for all people? One look at the current state of the world's health would suggest so. Nearly 1000 million people – almost one-fifth of the world's population – are caught up in a desperate daily struggle for survival, a continuous battle with poverty, malnutrition, disease and the energy-sapping prospect of little hope for improvement in the future. The majority of these people live in the rural areas and urban slums of the *least developed countries*, the poorest parts of the *developing world*. Of every 1000 children born into poverty in these countries, 125 will die within a year and another 80 will die before their fifth birthday. The average life expectancy of a child in the least developed countries is only 45–50 years, compared with 72–77 years in the *industrialised countries*.

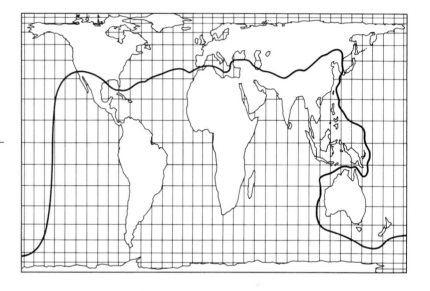

Most deaths in developing countries are the result of *infectious diseases* which are passed on from one person to another by bacteria, viruses, or parasites such as worms. Amongst these killer diseases are the common ailments of childhood, such as measles, diphtheria and polio, which have been effectively eradicated or brought under control in the industrialised world through immunisation programmes and improvements in living conditions. Over four and a half million children die each year – or more than 12,000 *each day* – from diarrhoeal infections in the developing world; on average, each child suffers three severe attacks of diarrhoea per year in their first four years of life. Disease is so widespread that it becomes an everyday occurrence: about one-tenth of a lifetime is likely to be seriously affected by disease. By contrast, in the industrialised world, the majority of deaths are caused by *degenerative diseases* such as coronary heart disease – alone accounting for about half of all deaths – and cancers. As life expectancy has increased, so too has the incidence of chronic degenerative disease. Also on the increase in industrialised countries are the numbers of people suffering from mental illness and from conditions relating to alcohol and drug

The children of the 1990s.

142 million children were born into the world in 1990. The chart presents this huge number as just 100 children and gives a schematic overview of what will happen to them.

100 born

| 12 | | 88 |

94 surviving to age one

| 12 | | 82 |

91 surviving to age five

| 12 | | 79 | → of which 28 are malnourished

85 starting primary school

| 12 | | 73 |

55 finishing primary school

| 11 | | 44 |

32 finishing secondary school

| 9 | | 23 |

☐ Industrialised world

▨ Developing world

abuse. During the 1980s a new and potentially devastating threat to health emerged: AIDS. The World Health Organisation has warned that during the 1990s the estimated number of people infected with HIV – the virus that causes AIDS – could rise from 5 million to over 30 million. So far, the majority of known cases of full-blown AIDS have occurred in North America and Western Europe, but the rapid increase in HIV infection in the highly populated countries of Africa and Asia is an alarming trend.

With such a catalogue of ill-health and disease throughout the world one might be tempted to question whether any progress at all has been made towards the goal of health for all by the year 2000. The statistics presented above, of course, need to be put into context. The proportion of children born who live beyond five years has increased substantially since 1950: from 65% to nearly 80% in the least developed countries, from 70% to 95% in other parts of the developing world, and from 92% to 99% in the industrialised countries. Average life expectancy at birth has risen appreciably: in China, for example, it is now 70 years (the same level as in the USA in the late 1950s) as against only 45 years in 1950, whilst in Africa as a whole it has risen from 38 to 51 years over the same period. Great progress has also been made worldwide in the immunisation of children against diphtheria, tuberculosis and polio; smallpox, which once infected 10-15 million people each year, was finally eradicated in 1977 thanks to a sustained vaccination programme co-ordinated

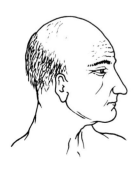

Progress in health care 1960–90

	1960	1990
Average life expectancy (in years)		
Least developed countries	38	50
Other developing countries	50	66
Industrialised countries	69	76
Average infant mortality*		
Least developed countries	185	116
Other developing countries	115	48
Industrialised countries	32	8

*No. of deaths of children under 1 year for every 1000 live births.
Source: Unicef.

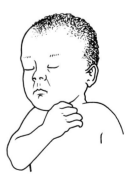

by WHO. These successful developments and trends in world health are even more encouraging when it is remembered that the world's population has increased from under 3 billion in 1950 to over 5 billion today. In general terms, more and more people are living longer, healthier lives.

Healthy, wealthy and wise?

'The first wealth is health.'
Ralph Waldo Emerson.

As with all statistics, figures on world health cover up as much as they reveal.

- *Why* do so many children in the developing world die of diseases which medical science has proven to be easily preventable?
- *Why* is the average life expectancy of an African some twenty-five years less than that of a European?
- *Why* do so many people in industrialised countries die of degenerative diseases which are relatively unknown in other parts of the world?

Answers to such questions will not be found by looking at statistics on health alone. The state of a person's – or a nation's – health is deeply entwined with so many social, political, economic and environmental factors. Just as it is impossible for a doctor to fully understand why a patient has developed cancer without exploring that person's living conditions, lifestyle and emotional state, so it is equally pointless to attempt any explanation of world health without an analysis of the relationship between health and wealth, the provision of basic needs such as food, water and housing, the availability of natural and technological resources, access to education, health and welfare services, and so on. In this book, health is centre stage, under the spotlight; but to appreciate the whole play, we must take account of the supporting cast. The remainder of this chapter introduces the other players whilst the succeeding chapters look at the role they each play.

The diagram below is a representation of the major influences on health. In the inner square are *basic needs* – the factors which are

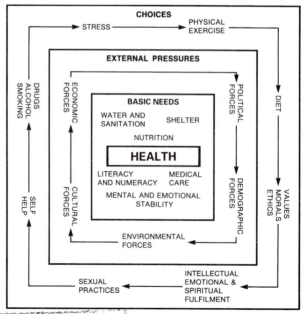

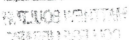

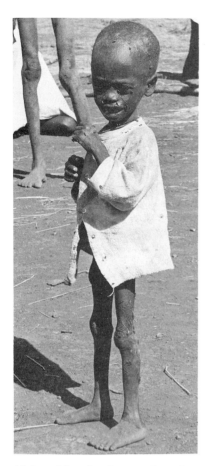

necessary for human survival and for minimum levels of dignity and self-respect. These might also be called *basic human rights*. The middle square represents the major *external pressures* on health. These are generally beyond the control of individuals, though in democratic societies they are shaped to some extent through the decisions of voters at the ballot box. As a result of such external pressures, some people's basic needs are met whilst other people have to struggle for survival. The outer square contains some key *choices* that individuals can make concerning the purpose and quality of their lives. Not all choices, of course, are open to all individuals because of constraints imposed by the external pressures; those people whose basic needs are barely met will have very few choices. The diagram gives a *holistic* view of health, in which the health of each person is seen to be related to the health of the society and of the planet. These connections will be explored fully in Chapter 9.

Basic needs

- *nutrition* Hundreds of millions of people in the developing world are undernourished. This impairs their ability to work and to learn and lowers their resistance to disease. Whereas the average daily energy supply for each person in the industrialised world is about 3450 calories – far in excess of actual need – it is barely 2000 calories per person in the least developed countries. In Africa, levels of nutrition have *declined* over the last twenty years. Overnutrition, or an excess of the wrong type of food, is a health problem in many parts of the industrialised world.
- *water and sanitation* Access to a safe water supply and effective disposal of sewage are prerequisites for health: about half of the world's most common diseases are transmitted by contaminated water. It is estimated that 25–35% of the world's population still lacks these basic facilities, despite the considerable progress made during the International Drinking Water Supply and Sanitation Decade, 1981–90.

Malnutrition, inadequate housing and poor sanitation are principal causes of ill-health in the developing world.

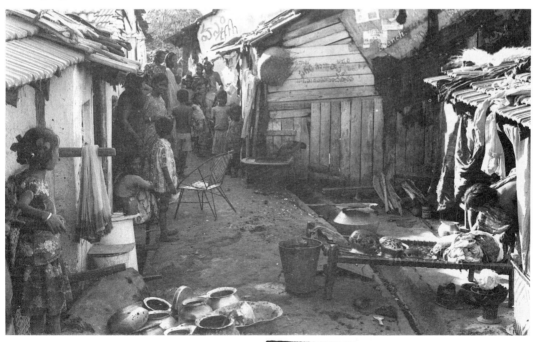

- *shelter* Homelessness is not only a developing-world problem; the streets of New York City are 'home' for some 50,000 people. The bright lights and job prospects in cities everywhere lure the poor and the unemployed, who are then forced to live on the streets or in urban slums in crowded conditions which are both degrading and ripe for disease. By the year 2000 about half of the world's people will be living in cities.
- *medical care* Trained medical personnel and medical supplies are unequally distributed throughout the world. Whilst there is on average one doctor for every 600 people in the industrialised world, there is one for 17,000 people in the least developed countries. Within countries, too, there is great disparity in medical provision between urban and rural areas – up to ten times as many people for each doctor in the country as in the city.
- *literacy and numeracy* Basic education is of major importance for health in that it enables people to understand their problems and to take responsibility for their own health. For women it is particularly crucial, for they carry the burden of the family's health – and yet an estimated 65% of the 900 million illiterate people in the world are women. More girls than boys are kept away from school so that they can help with domestic tasks.
- *mental and emotional stability* One-sixth of all people are mentally ill – twice as many women as men – but this form of suffering receives relatively little publicity and even less medical support: 90% of the developing world has virtually no mental health care. At the other end of the spectrum, mental illness has become 'fashionable' in some industrialised countries: in the USA there are now more mental health workers than police officers.

External pressures
- *economic forces* You don't have to be wealthy to be healthy, but it helps! Countries with a high *GNP* tend to have healthier people with longer life expectancies than countries with a low GNP, and the poor within each country are likely to be less healthy than the rich. The higher the GNP, the greater is the priority afforded to health expenditure: industrialised countries spend nearly 5% of

GNP: Gross National Product, the usual way of assessing the relative wealth of a country. It is a rough guide, arrived at by estimating the total annual value of all goods and services provided by a nation. It is then expressed as a *per capita* (per head) figure by dividing the total value by the country's population. This figure represents a guide to *economic wealth*, not necessarily to *quality of life*. For example, goods that are socially or environmentally destructive – such as armaments or pollutants – all contribute to GNP.

Government expenditure: selected countries

	Expenditure* on:		
	Health	Education	Defence
Pakistan	1	3	30
Somalia	1	2	38
India	2	3	19
Israel	4	10	27
Mozambique	5	10	35
Botswana	6	18	8
Zimbabwe	8	23	16
Australia	10	7	9
Nicaragua	11	9	50
UK	13	2	13
USA	13	2	25
Costa Rica	17	13	3
France	21	8	6

*As a percentage of total government expenditure, 1986–90.
Source: Unicef.

GNP on health compared with less than 2% spent by developing countries. Economic pressures are also exerted by the activities of multinational companies. Twenty major drug companies, all based in the industrialised world, account for over half of total world sales in drugs.

● *political forces* Many decisions about health expenditure are influenced by local and national politics. Different political systems finance and organise health services in different ways depending on whether the state or the individual is seen as having primary responsibility for paying for health care. Whatever the system, decisions taken by governments directly affect the health of individual citizens: those developing countries which allocate a high proportion of GNP to health care, such as Costa Rica and Cuba, tend to have longer-living and healthier people. Within countries, however, health care is not always equally available to all people.

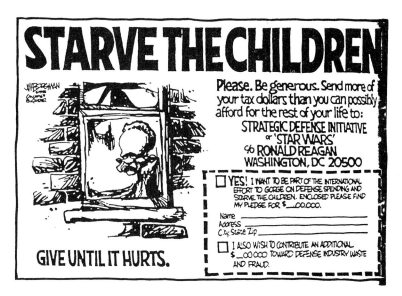

An American cartoonist's view of the effect of excessive spending on defence.

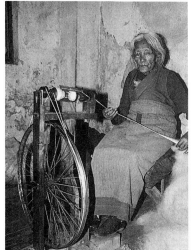

As health care in the developing world improves more people live into old age, like this woman in Darjeeling, India.

● *demographic forces* More people inevitably means that more resources for health care are needed, particularly in the developing world, where the rise in world population is concentrated. Advances in health care add to the burden by reducing the death rate and lengthening lives. In the long term, however, it has been shown that sustained improvement in the quality of their lives encourages people to have smaller families. Changes in the age structure of the population are likely to affect the pattern of disease. In 1980 more than half of the 260 million people aged over 65 lived in the industrialised world; by the year 2000 almost three-fifths of the estimated 400 million elderly will be in developing countries.

● *environmental forces* Health and the environment are deeply interconnected. Polluted air and water are responsible for the transmission of major infectious diseases; many degenerative diseases, particularly cancers, are thought to be attributable in part to environmental factors. The struggle to find diminishing natural resources such as firewood and water forces people to move to urban areas, thereby adding to the health problems of the cities.

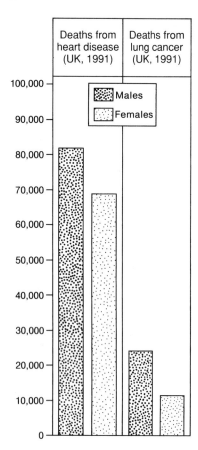

Deaths from heart disease (UK, 1991)	Deaths from lung cancer (UK, 1991)

Since 1950 there has been a substantial increase in deaths from lung cancer (90% due to smoking) in the industrialised world. Heart disease remains the biggest killer, despite a recent decline in deaths in many rich countries. A 1991 survey in England found that only 12% of men and 11% of women were free from the four main risk factors for heart disease – smoking, high blood pressure, high cholesterol level and lack of physical activity.

The pressures exerted by a person's living and working environment, including levels of stress, anxiety and powerlessness, can have a significant influence on mental and physical health.

● *cultural forces* Attitudes and beliefs have a powerful effect on health. Traditional practices such as female circumcision (see p. 61), which is known to cause severe medical problems, are maintained because of the strength of the belief on which they are based. Cultural and religious attitudes towards fertility and contraception can determine the number and spacing of children in a family, even where additional births may put the family's health at risk. A positive attitude towards oneself has been shown to have a beneficial effect on mental and physical health – a theory which has been part of Chinese medical practice for thousands of years.

Choices

For many people these are not real choices at all. *Diet* only becomes a matter of choice once more than enough food of the right quality is available; *physical exercise* is not an option for those whose bodies are emaciated by disease or malnutrition; high levels of *stress* can only be reduced by those who have sufficient control over their own lives. Real choices can only be made by those who fully understand the consequences of their actions. In many developing countries, where basic needs are not fully met, *smoking*, *alcohol* and *drug abuse* are on the increase because educational campaigns warning of their dangers do not reach much of the illiterate population. The spread of AIDS is much more difficult to contain in Africa than in North America for similar reasons.

An increasing number of people, particularly in the industrialised world, are in a position to make choices about the quality of their lives and their health. The last twenty years have seen a tremendous growth in *self-help* movements of all kinds – groups of people taking responsibility for their own health problems rather than seeking the advice of 'experts'. With ever-increasing knowledge about the dangers of drug abuse, of overeating, of certain sexual practices, health-related choices are becoming more numerous – though not necessarily any easier to make, as the very high incidence of death from coronary heart disease and lung cancer demonstrates. The health of a person, like the health of a nation, depends ultimately upon the priority it is given. Parts Two and Three of this book explore in detail some priorities in health care around the world and the choices open to individuals. In the next chapter we shall look at the major diseases and disabilities which afflict the world's people, so as to better understand the nature of ill-health.

2   Disease and disability

The causes of disease

Amongst any group of teenagers alive in Britain in the 1870s there would probably have been someone who had lost a young relative or friend as a result of a common childhood illness, such as measles, diphtheria or whooping cough. Today, death from these diseases is a rarity in the industrialised world and most children suffer only a few days' discomfort if they contract such a disease at all. Vaccinations against the six major childhood illnesses – the other three are polio, tuberculosis (TB) and tetanus – are now widely available. It would be misleading, however, to imply that *immunisation* has been the major cause of this improvement in children's health over the past hundred years. It has certainly helped but, as the graphs below show, the number of deaths from these diseases had declined sharply before vaccinations were introduced. Better housing, nutrition and education were of far greater significance.

The causes of any disease are many and complex, incorporating not only a 'disease agent' – such as a virus or bacteria – but also the

Immunisation is the practice of giving medicine, usually in the form of an injection, in order to prevent or reduce the severity of a disease. A *vaccine* is the medicine used in immunisation.

Decline in infectious diseases in the industrialised world.

Substantial health improvements have occurred mainly due to better public sanitation, housing and nutrition. Medical intervention has only significantly affected death rates since the 1940s.

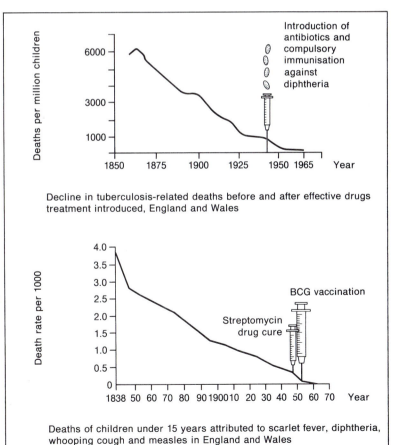

Decline in tuberculosis-related deaths before and after effective drugs treatment introduced, England and Wales

Deaths of children under 15 years attributed to scarlet fever, diphtheria, whooping cough and measles in England and Wales

physical and mental make-up of a sick person, their lifestyle and environment and their access to medical resources and information. Not all people infected with a disease agent become ill. For every 400 children infected with the polio virus, only one becomes paralysed. Whilst measles is a mild illness in the industrialised world, it is a major killer of African children. In the developing world, many people have little hope of preventing or controlling disease because their basic needs are never adequately met. Poverty entraps them in a vicious cycle of disease and disability which no amount of medicine alone can cure.

The story of Luis

Luis lived with his family in the small village of Platanar, 11 kilometres by dirt road from the town of San Ignacio, Mexico. In San Ignacio there is a health centre staffed by a doctor and several nurses, who run a vaccination programme. When Luis was four the health team came by jeep to Platanar, but after giving children the first of a series of vaccinations they never returned. Perhaps they were discouraged because many parents and children refused to co-operate; also, the road to Platanar is very dusty and hot. A local midwife went to San Ignacio, offering to take the vaccine back to the village and complete the series, so that the children would be fully protected against common diseases, including tetanus. The doctor refused, arguing that the children's lives would be put at risk unless the vaccination was carried out by someone with formal training.

Three years later Luis stepped on a long thorn whilst taking a bucket of food scraps to feed the family's pigs. He had bare feet because the sandals he normally wore had broken and were too worn out to repair. Luis' father, a poor farmer who had to give half his maize harvest as rent for the land he farmed, could not afford new sandals for his son. Luis pulled the thorn from his foot and limped home.

Nine days later the muscles in Luis' leg grew stiff and he had trouble opening his mouth. The following day he began to have spasms in which all the muscles in his body suddenly tightened and his back and neck bent backwards. The village midwife at first called his illness 'congestion' and recommended a herbal tea. But when the spasms got worse she suggested that Luis' parents take him to the health centre in San Ignacio. The family managed to borrow 500 pesos and paid one of the big landowners in Platanar to drive to San Ignacio in his truck. He charged them 300 pesos – much higher than the usual price.

At the health centre they waited for two hours. When they finally saw the doctor he at once diagnosed the illness as tetanus. He explained that Luis was in grave danger and needed injections of tetanus antitoxin; these were very expensive and, in any case, he did not have any. They would need to take Luis to the city of Mazatlan, 100 kilometres away.

The parents despaired. They had barely enough money left to pay the bus fare to Mazatlan. If their son died, how would they get his body back to the family graveyard in Platanar? So they thanked the doctor, paid his modest fee and took the afternoon bus back home.

Two days later, after great suffering, Luis died.

Source: D. Werner and B. Bower, *Helping Health Workers Learn,* Hesperian Foundation.

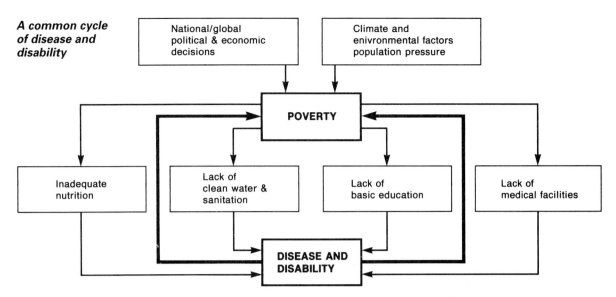

A common cycle of disease and disability

'The story of Luis', used in the training of health workers in Mexico, relates a complex but common chain of causes and events leading to the death of a child. It is easy to lay the blame at the door of the health team, the landowner or even the parents, but they are all part of a *global system* which keeps hundreds of millions of people in constant poverty; a system in which the policies and decisions of national governments – including those of industrialised countries – and international agencies play a significant role. Medical cures or preventive measures, such as vaccines, are important but they are only part of the solution that will save the lives of children like Luis. In Part Two we look at the economic and political factors that control the provision of health care and thereby decide the fate of many millions of people.

No fifth birthday

The table below shows how many children will die before they are five, in selected countries.

Mozambique	1 out of every 3
Ethiopia	1 out of every 4
Cambodia	1 out of every 5
Pakistan	1 out of every 6
Ghana	1 out of every 7
Peru	1 out of every 8
Honduras	1 out of every 9
Indonesia	1 out of every 10
Iran	1 out of every 15
Colombia	1 out of every 20
China	1 out of every 25
Poland	1 out of every 50
USA	1 out of every 75
UK	1 out of every 100
Netherlands	1 out of every 125
Japan	1 out of every 150

Source: Unicef

The diseases of poverty

1 Common childhood illnesses
One-quarter of all deaths in the world occur among children under five. 99% of all child deaths occur in developing countries. Further countless millions of children are physically or mentally disabled through disease. The real tragedy is that the vast majority of childhood illnesses can be prevented or contained by relatively low-cost measures such as immunisation, antibiotics and oral rehydration therapy (ORT).

Diarrhoea is the single largest cause of death. This infection, mostly the result of water-borne bacteria or viruses, causes severe dehydration and can kill rapidly. Oral rehydration salts, a simple mixture of salt and sugar in water which helps combat the dehydration, can save many of these lives. Since its introduction by the World Health Organisation in 1980, ORT is now used by one-third of the developing world's families, saving an estimated one million lives each year.

Measles accounts for half of the 3 million deaths each year which could be prevented by immunisation. Measles is also one of the major causes of malnutrition in children and severely weakens their bodies' resistance to other illnesses.

40,000 children die every day from malnutrition and infection.

Mother's health	Oral rehydration	Immunization	Breastfeeding
2m. children a year would be saved if their mothers had extra food during pregnancy	A mixture of salt, sugar and water could save 2m. diarrhoea deaths	Vaccines could save 5m. (measles alone kills 2m. a year)	1m. lives could be saved by elimination of unsuitable bottle feeding

Community health workers are people who work in their own towns and villages, having been given a training in basic health care and preventive medicine. The role of these workers is explored in Chapter 7.

'If we were to decide to observe a minute of silence for every person who died in 1982 owing to hunger-related causes, we would not be able to celebrate the advent of the 21st century.'
Fidel Castro, speaking in 1983.

What we eat

The World Health Organisation recommends a minimum daily adult calorie consumption of 2600 per head with variations for age, occupation and other factors. Yet average consumption in many poor countries falls far below this minimum, while that in rich countries is far in excess of it.

Acute respiratory infections, which include TB, diphtheria, whooping cough, bronchitis, pneumonia and influenza, can be prevented by immunisation or treated with antibiotics such as penicillin. Despite this knowledge, most *community health workers* have not been trained in the use of these medicines, often because of resistance from qualified doctors.

2 Deficiency diseases
Undernutrition – a critical shortage of food – and malnutrition – a deficiency of vital food elements – are a direct result of constant poverty. The Food and Agricultural Organisation (FAO) of the United Nations estimates that 500 million people (twice the population of the USA), of which 200 million are children, are literally starving to death whilst at least a further 300 million people are malnourished. Diseases that result from food deficiencies are rarely a direct cause of death but they are often a contributory factor as they increase the chances of infection, particularly amongst young

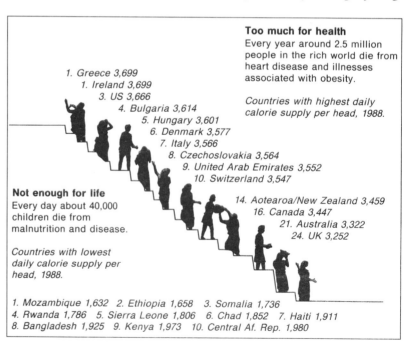

Too much for health
Every year around 2.5 million people in the rich world die from heart disease and illnesses associated with obesity.

Countries with highest daily calorie supply per head, 1988.

1. Greece 3,699
1. Ireland 3,699
3. US 3,666
4. Bulgaria 3,614
5. Hungary 3,601
6. Denmark 3,577
7. Italy 3,566
8. Czechoslovakia 3,564
9. United Arab Emirates 3,552
10. Switzerland 3,547
14. Aotearoa/New Zealand 3,459
16. Canada 3,447
21. Australia 3,322
24. UK 3,252

Not enough for life
Every day about 40,000 children die from malnutrition and disease.

Countries with lowest daily calorie supply per head, 1988.

1. Mozambique 1,632   2. Ethiopia 1,658   3. Somalia 1,736
4. Rwanda 1,786   5. Sierra Leone 1,806   6. Chad 1,852   7. Haiti 1,911
8. Bangladesh 1,925   9. Kenya 1,973   10. Central Af. Rep. 1,980

children. Physical and mental development can also be severely retarded.

Marasmus, or *severe protein-calorie malnutrition (PCM)*, and *kwashiorkor* (a Swahili word meaning 'the disease which comes when the second child is at the breast') usually result from a lack of protein intake once an infant has been weaned from the breast. The 'starving child' pictures on television during a major famine are graphic and pitiful reminders of the impact of these diseases.

Vitamin-A deficiency is often called 'blinding malnutrition' because half a million children each year are blinded through a lack of vitamin-A-rich foods such as dairy products and green vegetables. Many more children suffer impaired vision or have less resistance to other infections due to the lack of this essential vitamin.

Iodine deficiency occurs in mountainous areas wherever high rainfall washes iodine from the soil. Its effects range from severe physical disability, such as goitre (swelling of the thyroid gland) and cretinism (incomplete development due to thyroid deficiency), to mental retardation and poor performance at work and school. Some 800 million people are at risk.

3 Parasitic diseases

Malnutrition, lack of clean water and poor sanitation provide ideal conditions for insect-borne parasites found only in the developing world. The diseases they cause, sometimes called 'tropical diseases', between them affect one-third of the world's population. Parasitic infections have markedly decreased in countries that have succeeded in improving social and environmental conditions.

Malaria remains one of the world's most serious diseases despite a 30-year eradication programme; some of the malaria-carrying mosquitoes have become increasingly resistant to the common anti-malarial medicines. The disease now kills 2 million people each year, with 100 million people afflicted by repeated attacks of pain and fever. Malaria infects about half of all African children under the age of three.

Schistosomiasis (sometimes called *bilharzia*), caused by a snail-borne parasite, is an energy-sapping disease affecting over 200 million people. The schistosome parasite is passed on to humans through washing, bathing and playing in infected water.

Onchocerciasis or *river blindness* is transmitted by black flies which breed near running water. The disease causes total blindness in more

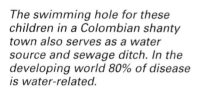

The swimming hole for these children in a Colombian shanty town also serves as a water source and sewage ditch. In the developing world 80% of disease is water-related.

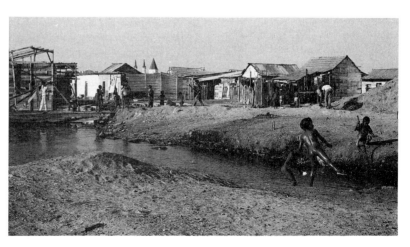

than 20% of the adult population in some parts of Africa. The spread of both schistosomiasis and onchocerciasis has increased because the snails and flies have found habitats in newly constructed dams and irrigation canals.

Ancylostomiasis (hookworm), ascariasis (roundworm) and *trichuriasis (whipworm)* make up the world's most common disease group, affecting one-third of the population. These three parasitic worms, often found in the same person, live off their host's blood after entering the body through the feet (hookworm) or the mouth via contaminated food and water (roundworm and whipworm). The diseases are rarely fatal but can cause severe anaemia and apathy.

Guinea worm disease is caused by drinking water contaminated by microscopic water fleas containing Guinea worm larvae. Once in the human body the worm grows up to a metre long, eventually emerging twelve months later through a painful skin ulcer. The disease causes crippling pain and general body weakness in 20 million people in Africa and Asia, and a further 140 million are at risk.

The diseases of affluence

The *infant mortality rate* is the annual number of deaths of infants under one year of age per 1000 live births. This statistic is commonly used as an indicator of a country's level of development.

It is no coincidence that the patterns of disease and causes of premature death in the wealthier, industrialised countries are vastly different from those found in the developing world. Yet less than 150 years ago, the *infant mortality rate* in Liverpool at the height of immigration to the city caused by the Irish potato famine was 229 per thousand births – far higher than in most cities in the developing world today. As one historian observed, 'the inevitable result of this influx of desperately poor people was a massive outbreak of typhus accompanied by epidemics of smallpox, measles, scarlet fever, tuberculosis and in 1849 the devastating Asiatic Cholera'. The underlying causes of these infant deaths were very similar to the factors which now contribute to the high mortality rate in cities such as Calcutta, Nairobi and São Paulo: poverty, overcrowding, poor sanitation and inadequate nutrition. The wealth created since the industrial revolution has largely eradicated these social and environmental causes of disease throughout the industrialised world, where the average infant mortality rate is now under ten. The scale of premature death and disease in the rich world is therefore much lower than in developing countries. Affluence and industrialisation, however, have brought about new health problems of which the most common are heart disease and cancer.

Heart disease accounts for nearly 50% of all deaths in the industrialised world. Heart attacks are fatal for half of all sufferers and cause disability for many others. A heart attack occurs if blood cannot flow freely in one or both coronary arteries due to a build-up of fatty material containing cholesterol in the artery wall. The major causes of heart disease are connected with diet and lifestyle: obesity, a high-fat diet, smoking, lack of regular exercise, and stress. Prior to the industrial revolution, heart disease was rare in Britain. The demand for energy-rich food in the fast-growing manufacturing cities prompted farmers to fatten up their cows, lambs and pigs, thereby contributing to a major epidemic. Britain now has the highest rate of heart disease in the world.

Cancer causes 20% of deaths, and affects nearly 1 in 3 people, in the rich world. Lung cancer is the biggest killer despite a decreasing trend in many countries due to a reduction in smoking. Breast cancer is the major concern for women, affecting 1 in 12 British women and causing 300 deaths per week – the highest mortality rate in the world for this type of cancer. Some cancers, such as those of the stomach and bowel, are occurring less in younger people, probably due to changes in diet and food preservation. Cancer treatments – surgery, drugs and radiotherapy – are helping to reduce death rates overall, but new dangers are emerging. An increase in skin cancer is attributed to damage to the ozone layer, allowing harmful ultraviolet radiation to reach the earth. Environmental and chemical factors are thought to be contributory causes in 4 out of 5 cancers.

It is important to remember that poverty still exists – and may be on the increase – in the industrialised world and, conversely, there is an affluent minority in the developing world. Disease patterns tend to reflect social circumstance. Within the city of Sheffield the chance of dying from heart disease is three times as great in some districts compared with others. A recent British government survey concluded that infant deaths regarded as 'preventable' were three times as likely to occur amongst children born into Social Class V than into Social Class I. The infant death rate is also much higher than average amongst certain ethnic minority groups. The Child Poverty Action Group calculates that more than 2 million children in the UK are now living below the poverty line, and serious concern has been expressed about the poor nutrition of children in low-income families who are no longer entitled to free school meals. Another worrying statistic from the 1980s is a rising trend in cases of TB – a good general indicator of standards of diet, housing and health.

Social health of children and youth, USA, 1970–87

The graph shows changes in the Index of Social Health for Children and Youth in the United States. The index is a composite measure, on a 0 to 100 scale, of performance in six critical areas: infant mortality, child abuse, child poverty, teenage suicide, drug abuse, and high-school drop-outs.

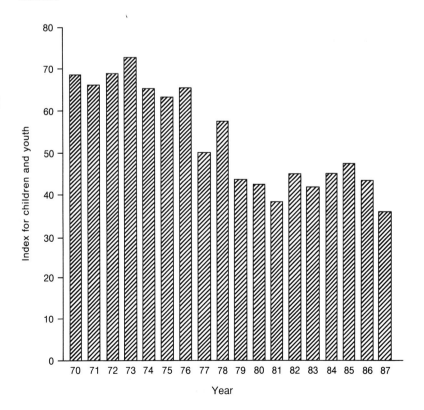

As industrialisation and Western culture spread into the developing world, so, too, do the 'diseases of affluence'. Thirty years ago in Jamaica a heart-attack patient would have been considered a novelty, to be shown off to student doctors. Today, a serious epidemic of heart disease is predicted in many countries of the Caribbean, largely due to a dramatic increase in the fat content of the diet. Over half of all Caribbean women, and more than a quarter of all men, are reported to be obese. In much calypso and reggae music, being fat is associated with wealth and success; being thin is an uncomfortable reminder of the malnutrition which, not too long ago, led to the death of many Caribbean children.

Heart disease is responsible for more than one-third of all deaths in newly industrialised nations such as Singapore, Kuwait and Venezuela. Smoking is the principal cause of a rapid increase in heart disease in India and Pakistan and also accounts for recent high death rates from lung cancer in China and Hong Kong. Of the estimated annual total of 6 million new cases of cancer in the world, more than half now arise in developing nations. (Apart from smoking, however, the causes are different from those in the rich world, being mainly due to viruses, inadequate diet and lack of screening facilities.) The spread of degenerative diseases has prompted governments in some poorer nations to spend vastly disproportionate amounts of their health budgets on high-tech facilities, such as heart surgery units, rather than committing that money to fighting the infectious diseases which still afflict the majority of their people.

Cancer as a whole is increasing slowly, with the exception of lung cancer, which is increasing at almost epidemic proportions in many parts of the world. The global mortality rate for cancers is 4.3 million annually, of which 2.3 million occur in the developing world.

Cancer by region

Most common cancer types ranked within regions (1986)

Region	Sex	1 Cancer	Total cases	2 Cancer	Total cases	3 Cancer	Total cases
Latin America	♂	Stomach	28,000	Lung	25,000	Prostate	19,000
	♀	Breast	49,000	Cervix	44,000	Stomach	17,000
Africa	♂	Liver	43,000	Lymphatic	20,000	Mouth	13,000
	♀	Cervix	37,000	Breast	27,000	Lymphatic	12,000
China	♂	Stomach	128,000	Oesophagus	109,000	Liver	81,000
	♀	Cervix	137,000	Stomach	68,000	Oesophagus	59,000
India and other Asia	♂	Mouth	97,000	Lung	62,000	Stomach	43,000
	♀	Cervix	141,000	Breast	95,000	Mouth	48,000
UK*	♂	Lung	30,000	Prostate	10,000	Bladder	7,000
	♀	Breast	24,000	Lung	11,000	Colon	9,000

*UK figures (1984) included for comparison to indicate the pattern typical of industrialised countries.
Source: New Internationalist, August 1989.

Mental illness and disability

The WHO goal of 'health for all by the year 2000' incorporates mental as well as physical health. Recent WHO reports suggest, however, that there is a threat of a *pandemic* of mental illness across the world. As populations grow and lives are prolonged, the number

Pandemic: an epidemic which spreads over a wide area.

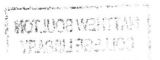

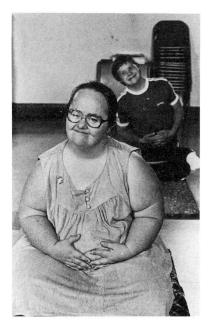

A yoga class for mentally disabled people in Sydney, Australia. Permanent mental disability affects over 100 million people.

of people at high risk of developing mental disorders also increases. One person out of every six is affected by mental illness at some time in their lives and yet only about 1% of world health expenditure goes towards mental health, mostly spent in the industrialised world.

There are two main categories of mental illness, neuroses and psychoses.

Neuroses, accounting for 4 out of 5 cases of mental illness, are relatively mild disorders often connected with stress and resulting in anxiety and phobias. Treatment is commonly provided through tranquillising or mood-altering drugs, many of which can be obtained without a doctor's prescription and can be addictive.

Psychoses are severe mental disorders, such as schizophrenia, depression and dementia, from which patients suffer delusions, hallucinations and acute emotional disturbance. Many sufferers are admitted to mental hospitals for treatment through powerful drugs and electro-convulsive therapy (ECT), which involves passing a mild electric current through part of the brain.

Mental illness can also result from damage to the brain caused by bacterial and parasitic infections, malnutrition, alcohol and drug abuse. Permanent brain damage, particularly when present at birth or due to head injuries, is usually referred to as *mental disability* or *handicap*. Over 100 million people in the world, or 1 in 60, suffer from serious intellectual and emotional disabilities which limit their ability to learn and prevent them from leading a normal life.

But what is 'normal'? The line between 'sanity' and 'insanity' is very thin: behaviour that is regarded as 'abnormal' and 'socially unacceptable' in one society is tolerated in another. In Japan, the proportion of patients detained in mental hospitals without their consent is 100 times greater than in Europe. Mental illness is frequently cited by totalitarian governments as a reason for detaining people who oppose their viewpoint. There are disturbing variations, too, in the rates of mental illness between social and ethnic groups. The impact of racism is believed to explain the over-representation of black and Irish immigrants in UK mental hospitals, and of Maori and Polynesian peoples in New Zealand institutions. Amongst Australian Aborigines, the high rate of death by suicide – virtually unknown before European colonisation – has been attributed to the acute bewilderment experienced by black Australians at the loss of their land, on which they depended for spiritual as well as physical well-being.

Such examples suggest that social cohesion – the ability of individuals and communities to live in harmony with each other – and social justice are basic requirements for mental health. The predicted pandemic of mental illness may be directly related to the spread of Western industrialisation, which commonly puts the individual before the community and values competition over co-operation. It has been suggested that the distinction we make between 'mental' and 'physical' illness is another product of Western industrial thinking, which likes to separate and classify things rather than seeking the relationship between them. Doctors in 18th-century England took a much more *holistic* view of health in which mind, body and spirit were regarded as deeply connected. This view is becoming fashionable again in many Western, post-industrial societies, leading to a growth in 'alternative medicine'. This will be explored in Chapter 8.

Priorities in the 1990s

At the World Summit for Children in September 1990 the following seven targets were agreed for the decade up to the year 2000:
- 33% reduction in the under-five child mortality rates
- 50% reduction in maternal mortality rates (death of women in pregnancy or childbirth)
- 50% reduction of severe and moderate malnutrition among children under five
- access to safe water and sanitation for all families
- access to basic education for all children
- 50% reduction in the adult illiteracy rate and achievement of equal educational opportunities for women
- protection of children in especially difficult circumstances, particularly in war zones

These goals for the world's children reflect most of the priorities for health care in the developing world, designed to reduce the number

State of health indicators

The table below summarises the state of the world's health according to ten indicators. Countries are grouped using the Unicef Under-5 Mortality Rate (U5MR) scale (see note 1 below). The statistics (see note 2) clearly illustrate the close relationship between health, education and wealth.

Indicator	Very high U5MR countries[3]	High U5MR countries[4]	Middle U5MR countries[5]	Low U5MR countries[6]
Infant mortality rate	118	67	27	9
Life expectancy (at birth)	49	61	70	76
Access to health services (% of population)	46	75	82	100
Access to safe water (% of population)	44	52	83	100
Daily per capita calorie supply (as % of requirements)	91	109	122	129
Population annual growth rate (1980–89)	2.9	2.8	2.0	0.5
Adult literacy rate: male/female	45/19	73/55	88/85	97/90
Primary school completion (% of grade 1 enrolment)	50	66	81	95
GNP per capita (US $)	295	830	1725	12575
Radio/television sets (no. per 1000 population)	99/6	145/54	261/114	610/368

Notes:
[1] The Under-5 Mortality Rate is the annual number of deaths of children under 5 years of age per 1000 live births. It is, suggest Unicef, the single most accurate indicator of the health of a nation's children, and of society as a whole.
[2] The figures given on the chart represent the *median* values for each group of countries.
[3] This group includes 38 countries with a total population of 1511 million.
[4] This group includes 31 countries with a total population of 886 million.
[5] This group includes 28 countries with a total population of 1894 million.
[6] This group includes 32 countries with a total population of 889 million.
Source: The State of the World's Children 1990 and 1991, Unicef/Oxford University Press.

of premature deaths caused by poverty, malnutrition and infection. Some of these goals are equally relevant in industrialised nations: the US government's national health targets for the year 2000 include significant reductions in infant and maternal mortality rates, particularly amongst Black and Hispanic groups. The achievement of such targets by the end of the decade does not require sophisticated knowledge or technology. What is needed, however, may be more difficult to obtain: a commitment on the part of all governments to ensure that the world's poorest people have access to adequate food and shelter, clean water and basic education.

It is likely that over 90% of the world's spending on health will *not* be devoted to achieving these goals in the 1990s. The priorities for funding will probably be the treatment of heart disease, cancers and other degenerative diseases, mental illness and AIDS – the conditions which directly affect the health of people living in the richer nations. Whilst acknowledging the importance of low-tech and low-cost approaches to health care in the South, the North continues to fund high-tech treatments using sophisticated surgery and expensive drugs. Are the 'diseases of affluence' only curable through the latest technology? Or would it be more beneficial – and a lot cheaper – to pay more attention to the underlying emotional, social and environmental conditions which cause illness? How can such expenditure in the North be justified under a policy of 'health for *all*' when disease is so much more common – and more devastating – in the South? And anyway, by putting so much faith in the ability of doctors and scientists to find cures for disease, is there not a danger of forgetting that health problems may well be directly related to personal lifestyles and emotional states? Such questions pose a major dilemma for the health care industry in the late 20th century. Part Two explores some of the principal arguments through looking in depth at some global crises which will question the effectiveness and the justice of health provision until well into the 21st century. Part Three looks at ways in which people in different parts of the world have attempted to find their own answers to these questions.

3   Smoking: a preventable epidemic?

'If tobacco were to be introduced today as a new product, it would not meet the safety standards of any country and would be outlawed.'
Dr Halfdan Mahler, formerly WHO Director General.

Cigarettes – legal but deadly

In 1978 the British charity War on Want published a report entitled *Tobacco and the Third World: Tomorrow's Epidemic?*. 'The harmful effects of cigarette smoking', the report suggested, 'are largely the result of the development this century of the modern cigarette. Many of the diseases associated with smoking have been widespread for only a few generations – mainly in the rich countries of Europe and North America. For the poorer developing countries, smoking-related disease is still tomorrow's epidemic.' There is now mounting evidence to show that 'tomorrow's epidemic' has arrived in parts of the developing world, so adding to the already considerable burden of dealing with malnutrition and infectious diseases.

Since 1971, all advertisements for cigarettes have carried a health warning and they have gradually increased in severity. All cigarette packs are now required to carry two health warnings in addition to information about tar and nicotine yields. A health warning also appears on cigars and other tobacco products as well as on tobacco advertising.

Smoking kills

Smoking causes cancer

Smoking causes heart disease

Smoking when pregnant harms your baby

'Cigarettes are the only legal product that, when used as intended, cause death.'
Louis W. Sullivan, US Secretary of Health and Human Services.

'Tobacco kills two and a half million people a year worldwide: equivalent to two or three jumbo jet-loads a day.'
Dr John Roberts, WHO.

   In the industrialised world we have grown accustomed to the health warnings printed on cigarette packets and advertisements. Whilst there is evidence to suggest that such warnings and other anti-smoking publicity have contributed to a decline in smoking in Europe and North America, it is probably true that the real dangers of tobacco are not widely understood. What the health warnings fail to point out is that nicotine is one of the most addictive of all known drugs, more so than illegal drugs such as cannabis and LSD. Although nicotine by itself is relatively harmless, the concoction of chemicals and gases that go with it in a cigarette is potentially deadly, and every cigarette smoked is thought to contribute to the long-term damage of internal organs. There is now overwhelming evidence to support the view that smoking is responsible for 25% of all heart disease, 75% of bronchitis cases and 90% of lung cancers, as well as being associated with many other cancers. The short-term effects include increasing the severity of influenza, damaging the body's immune system, adversely affecting the foetus of a pregnant woman and diminishing athletic performance.

Recent research has highlighted the dangers of 'passive smoking' – the inhaling of cigarette smoke by non-smokers who live or work in a smoke-filled environment. The American Association for Cancer Research says that non-smoking women who live with a smoker have a 30-50% increased risk of developing lung cancer. A British study found that non-smoking children with two smoking parents had the equivalent nicotine in their bodies of someone who smoked seven cigarettes a week; and a Glasgow-based study concluded that passive smoking in Britain probably kills 500 people a year. The US Environmental Protection Agency puts tobacco smoke in the highest category of cancer-inducing substances, alongside asbestos (on which there are strict regulations for usage). As the evidence on the health risks of passive smoking mounts, enclosed public facilities such as theatres, community centres and transportation vehicles are increasingly becoming 'smoke-free zones'. In Belgium and Finland smoking is prohibited in all public places. Many private employers now forbid smoking in the workplace; the De Havilland company in Canada has been fined under the Occupational Health and Safety Act for dismissing an employee who refused to work in a tobacco-filled environment. This anti-smoking trend angers some civil liberty and pro-smoking groups, who reject the research evidence on passive smoking and argue that the prohibition of smoking is a denial of individual rights.

A Health Education Authority cartoon designed to inform children of the dangers of nicotine.

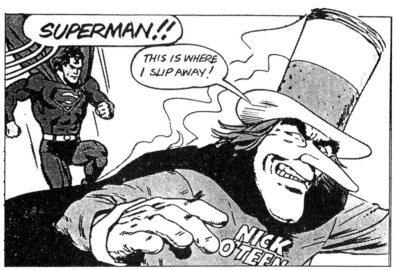

In addition to the dangers posed by cigarettes themselves, it seems that smoking is often the start of a chain of drug-taking practice. A survey of children in the UK found that 50% of children who were regular smokers had experimented with illegal drugs, compared with 2% of non-smokers; in Norway 33% of daily smokers aged 15–24 are involved in glue-sniffing, compared with 2% of non-smokers. The use of drugs and alcohol is also a contributory factor in many traffic accidents, a major cause of death and disability amongst young people.

The fashionable drug

Throughout history drugs have been used for their mind-expanding or hallucinogenic properties. In the Middle Ages witches in Europe were persecuted for their knowledge and use of plants such as mandrake and deadly nightshade. The Bohemians shocked Paris in the 1840s through their excessive use of a stimulant drug which 'made the sufferer tremulous, subject to fits of agitation and depression'. The drug was coffee. Until the end of the 19th century opium was as freely available in Britain as cigarettes are today. Romantic poets Baudelaire (who formed a hashish smokers' club) and W.B. Yeats (who took mescaline – a hallucinogen) are amongst the many writers and artists to have used drugs. During the Second World War, the American, British, German and Japanese armies were issued with amphetamines to keep them going. Today many formerly common drugs are illegal, whilst others – alcohol, caffeine, tobacco, tranquillisers – are consumed in vast quantities as acceptable means of coping with the pressures of everyday life. It seems that for many people drugs have become a necessary tool in their daily survival kit.

The habit of smoking, like many other forms of drug-taking, usually begins as a social activity. Pressure to 'be one of us' is likely to come from school friends, from brothers, sisters or parents, or from colleagues in the workplace. For many young people a cigarette is a status symbol, a sign of maturity and adulthood, a show of sophistication. Girls, in particular, believe that smoking helps them lose weight and look more attractive. The health warnings are ignored because the psychological and social advantages of being seen with a cigarette outweigh the unknown and far-off dangers to health. The grave danger of teenage smoking lies in the addictive power of tobacco. Statistics reveal that the younger a person starts to smoke, the greater is their expected loss of life – an average of eight years if smoking begins at 15, four years if at 25. If tobacco is not taken up in adolescence it rarely is in later life: as many as 90% of eventual smokers started before the age of 19. A survey of school students in the UK indicates that by the age of 15 more than 60% have tried smoking at least once or twice and that 25% of girls are regular smokers. Some 14 million British adults – about one-third of the adult population – are thought to be smokers.

The use of tobacco by young people is widespread in all parts of the world and is on the increase in developing countries, particularly amongst women. It is estimated that by the year 2000 there will be 2 million new lung cancer cases each year in these countries, double the present world total. In the industrialised world the number of women dying annually from lung cancer doubled between 1960 and 1980; since the mid-1980s lung cancer has overtaken breast cancer as the most common form of cancer in American women, a trend which is predicted for the UK by the year 2010.

Medical experts have suggested that tobacco is the greatest single cause of non-communicable disease and is likely to give rise to a world epidemic unless urgent preventive action is taken. The main impact of that epidemic will be felt in the developing world, where the annual consumption of cigarettes is rising by 3% each year. Unlike the major killer diseases which are the inevitable products of malnutrition and poverty, smoking causes self-inflicted illness. What are the factors which promote smoking-related disease? Why is

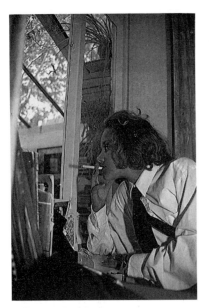

Sophisticated or stupid? Many young people take up smoking because of the image it creates.

'Among an average 1000 young men who smoke cigarettes regularly:
- about 1 will be murdered
- about 6 will be killed on the roads
- about 250 will be killed by tobacco'
British Medical Association.

Smoking prevalence among young people (ages as indicated) in selected countries.

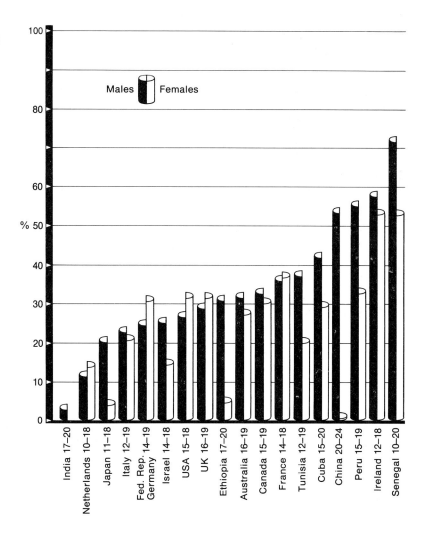

smoking becoming increasingly fashionable in developing countries at a time when hundreds of millions of people do not have enough money to buy food, clothes or medicines?

Tobacco is big business

Tobacco had been smoked by native Americans for centuries before the plant was brought back to Paris in about 1550 by Jean Nicot, the young French ambassador to Lisbon. Nicot, whose name survives in the word nicotine, made a fortune from the tobacco trade he established – a trade which has continued to thrive and now generates profits of $3000 million a year for the multinational companies involved. Cigarette consumption worldwide has more than doubled since 1960 even though it is now decreasing by 1% a year in the industrialised countries. Over the past 20 years, 40 million Americans and 5.5 million Canadians have given up smoking; in the last decade 10 million Britons kicked the habit. Faced with what appears to be a fast-growing anti-smoking trend in the industrialised world, tobacco companies have turned their attention – and their considerable marketing power – to the developing world.

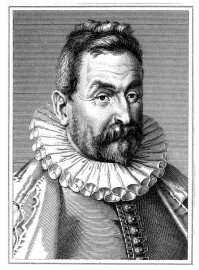

Jean Nicot, diplomat and tobacco importer.

27

The developing world's production of tobacco will have doubled between 1975 and 2000, generating vital income for these countries.

World tobacco production (farm–sales–weight)

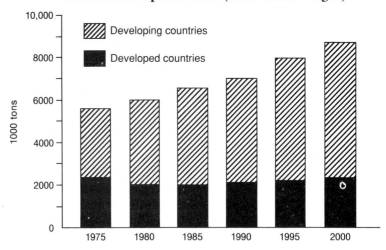

A key argument put forward by tobacco companies for maintaining the increase in cigarette consumption concerns the economic prosperity of developing countries, where over 75% of the world's tobacco crop is grown. According to David Walder, chief executive of the International Tobacco Growers' Association, 'too many decisions about tobacco are being taken without any thought given to the implications for the small farmers who are our members or to the economies of their countries'. About 90% of the 33 million people engaged in the tobacco industry are from developing countries. In Zimbabwe, one of the world's top four tobacco exporters, 6% of the population is dependent upon the industry; tobacco is the main generator of foreign exchange income in Malawi, one of the poorest countries in the world. This poses a dilemma for the World Health Organisation, which, whilst campaigning vigorously against smoking, also recognises the importance of economic prosperity to improving the health of people in the developing world.

The economic argument is, however, refuted by Dr Halfdan Mahler, WHO's former Director General. He maintains that such income 'is fool's gold, because the economic gains are more than cancelled out by premature deaths, medical bills, fires caused by careless smokers, and absenteeism and lost productivity associated with tobacco-related disease'. This point is most pertinent in those countries such as China – the world's largest producer and consumer of cigarettes – where the tobacco crop is grown for home use. Zimbabwe, on the other hand, currently exports about 98% of its tobacco to 80 countries worldwide, thereby generating much-needed income whilst avoiding, at present, the harmful effects of smoking. Yet it is to the developing countries that tobacco-exporting nations are increasingly having to turn as smoking declines in the industrialised world. The world looks set for an epidemic in which the poorest nations will need to sell their dangerous products to their own people or to other poor nations, thereby cancelling out some of the progress made towards 'health for all'. Behind this perverse arrangement is the wealth and power of the tobacco companies, which spend $2 billion a year in advertising their products, and the priorities of national governments, which reap considerable rewards from tobacco taxation.

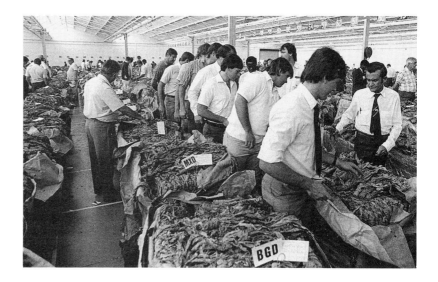

Tobacco being auctioned in Harare, Zimbabwe. This sales floor is the biggest of its kind in the world.

The politics of smoking

King James II of England declared smoking to be 'a custom loathsome to the eye, hateful to the nose, harmful to the brain, dangerous to the lungs'. That did not prevent him, however, from lowering the import duty on tobacco, which encouraged its consumption and increased the revenues due to him. Queen Elizabeth II is a non-smoker, as are most of the Royal Family; the Duke of Gloucester is Patron of the anti-smoking pressure group ASH and President of Parents Against Tobacco. Yet Benson and Hedges can still proudly display on cigarette packets a royal warrant as 'Purveyors of Cigars and Cigarettes to Her Majesty the Queen'. Where tobacco is concerned, double standards have a long and distinguished history.

In 1989/90 the UK government earned over £6000 million from taxes on tobacco products and spent about £7 million on campaigns and health warnings to discourage smoking. The annual cost to the National Health Service of caring for people with severe smoking-related illnesses is put at £500 million, though this figure does not take into account the medical care needed, and working days lost, by the millions of smokers (and non-smokers) who constantly suffer from the less severe effects of tobacco. Even so, from a purely economic standpoint it is easy to see why the UK government – like many other governments around the world – has moved very cautiously to discourage smoking. Although cigarette advertising on television was banned in 1964, the promotion of tobacco products in other ways is largely controlled not by law but by voluntary agreements between the government and the manufacturers.

A total ban in Europe on all publicity for tobacco products has been proposed by the European Commission, though opposed by three EC member countries – Germany, The Netherlands and the UK. Their opposition is a comfort to the tobacco industry, which, together with advertising and publishing companies, argues that such a ban would have a devastating effect not only on tobacco companies but also on the media and advertising industries. Most UK national newspaper supplements, one survey suggests, would lose

'So long as the UK government continues to rely on cosy agreements with the tobacco industry they will condemn hundreds of thousands of British men and women to disease and early deaths.'
David Pollock, Director, ASH.

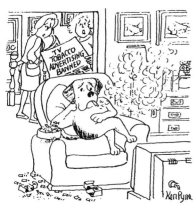

'I'm afraid it's come too late for the beagle we adopted'

This cartoonist reminds us that dogs have been used in medical experiments to test the effects of smoking cigarettes.

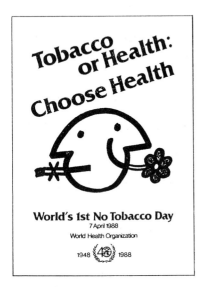

£3–4 million a year in advertising revenue; throughout Europe an estimated 16,000 jobs in the magazine industry could be lost and 2000 publications forced to close. The ban would also hit major sporting events which are presently sponsored by tobacco companies, whose names and logos could not be associated with sport. The tobacco industry claims that advertising does not encourage people to smoke but is merely concerned with establishing a smoker's loyalty to a particular brand. The anti-smoking lobby disagrees. David Pollock, Director of ASH (Action on Smoking and Health) points to evidence from Canada, Finland and New Zealand which shows a decline in tobacco consumption following an advertising ban.

In view of the downward trend in smoking in the industrialised world, the tobacco industry has been looking to developing countries to expand exports. According to tobacco economist Dan Stevens, 'it will require imagination and creativity to market tobacco in these markets'; nonetheless, he predicts a worldwide increase in tobacco use of about 2% a year over the next ten years. There can be little doubt that the multinational tobacco companies have the resources to mount very imaginative and effective marketing campaigns in the developing world; and that the image of prosperity and sophistication which cigarette advertising promotes will appeal to the poor and disadvantaged, despite the health warnings. At governmental level the economic argument for continued growth in the tobacco industry is summarised by the International Tobacco Growers' Association:

> *Without continuing substantial taxation proceeds from tobacco many First World countries will not be able to maintain their own health and welfare programmes; without the foreign exchange earnings from tobacco growing many developing countries would need very substantial development and emergency aid from First World countries to help ward off widespread economic and social hardship.*

Such are the economic and political mountains that the World Health Organisation still has to climb in order to eradicate smoking-related disease. WHO's slogan for the first 'No Tobacco Day' in 1988 was: *Tobacco or Health: Choose Health*. The choice, it seems, is not quite that simple.

4   AIDS: world health's greatest challenge

The short history of AIDS

In 1981 a new disease affecting gay men in America was first recognised by doctors working at the Centers for Disease Control in Atlanta, USA. The symptoms included forms of skin cancer and pneumonia which did not normally affect healthy people. Two years later a French doctor, Luc Montagnier, and an American, Robert Gallo, separately identified the virus which caused the disease. The virus has since become known as HIV (Human Immunodeficiency Virus) and the disease as AIDS (Acquired Immune Deficiency Syndrome).

Scientists now think that HIV became a new human virus more than a hundred years ago, possibly evolving from a monkey virus in Central Africa. It appears to have had little impact in Africa until increasing migration of men in search of work in the major cities led to changes in the pattern of sexual relationships. Other theories suggest that HIV originated in the USA – where most of the early AIDS victims were identified – and then spread to Africa, perhaps via Europe.

Research carried out in 1988 indicated three distinct patterns of HIV transmission in the world:

Pattern 1 – *Western Europe, North America, Latin America (urban areas), Australia and New Zealand*
Transmission mainly through sex between homosexual men and by drug users sharing needles. Male sufferers outnumbered females by 10 or 15 to 1.

Pattern 2 – *Central, Eastern and Southern Africa, parts of the Caribbean and Latin America*
Transmission mainly through heterosexual sex, transfusions of infected blood and from mother to unborn child. The ratio of infected males to females was 1 to 1.

Pattern 3 – *North Africa, Eastern Europe, Middle East, Pacific (excluding Australia and New Zealand)*
Transmission mainly through heterosexual and homosexual sex, probably introduced in the mid-1980s from contact with people in pattern areas 1 and 2.

At the time that research was carried out there were 75,000 reported cases of AIDS worldwide, a sixfold increase in just three years. Three years later, the total had reached nearly half a million and WHO predicted that there would be 12–18 million AIDS sufferers by the end of the century, with 30–40 million people being HIV infected. Furthermore, heterosexual intercourse had become the principal mode of HIV transmission in most parts of the world. It is the speed at which the disease is spreading, and its prevalence in all regions of the world, which makes AIDS unique amongst the present challenges to world health.

What is AIDS?

AIDS (Acquired Immune Deficiency Syndrome) is a disease in which the body's natural immune system, which fights infection, is seriously damaged.

AIDS is caused by the virus HIV (Human Immunodeficiency Virus). HIV infects T-cells, the body's main line of defence against all other infections.

Not everyone with HIV has AIDS. It is thought that 30-50% of people infected with HIV will eventually develop 'full-blown' AIDS. There can be a gap of up to 10 years from HIV infection to the emergence of AIDS symptoms. AIDS is nearly always fatal, but the time-lapse between diagnosis and death varies.

People with less serious AIDS symptoms are said to be suffering from ARC (AIDS-Related Complex).

Anyone infected with HIV can pass on the virus to others.

What happens to AIDS sufferers?

People with HIV infection may show no signs of disease for many years, though diagnosis can be made through a blood test. The commonest symptoms of AIDS and ARC include:

- swollen glands, especially in the neck and armpits
- profound fatigue, lasting for several weeks
- unexpected weight loss – more than 10 lbs in two months
- fever and night sweats, lasting for several weeks
- prolonged shortness of breath and a dry cough
- prolonged diarrhoea
- skin disease – pink or purple blotches.

Any of these symptoms may, however, be caused by other illnesses.

AIDS patients generally die from lack of resistance to common infections, from a form of cancer or from destruction of brain cells.

How is AIDS transmitted?

HIV is passed on when blood, semen or vaginal fluids from an infected person pass directly into another person's blood stream. This can only happen in a few ways:

- through sexual intercourse between a man and a woman or between men
- through the injection of infected blood, either by the use of unsterilised needles and syringes, or in blood transfusions where the blood has not been HIV tested
- from an infected mother to her unborn or new-born child and through breastfeeding.

THE MYTHS

AIDS

THE FACTS

How is AIDS not transmitted?

HIV is a weak virus that cannot survive for long outside the body. It cannot be spread by contact with an HIV infected person, other than in the ways stated above. The following practices do *not* constitute a risk of HIV infection (even if carried out by or with someone who has HIV): social kissing, caressing, love-bites, handling genitals; sneezing, sweating, sharing toilets, washing machines, cutlery or musical instruments; giving blood.

There is no risk from sexual intercourse between uninfected people.

Source: compiled from WHO and other sources.

How can AIDS be prevented?

At present there is no known cure for HIV infection. The risk of catching or passing on HIV can be reduced by:

- practising 'safer sex' – any sexual practice which minimises the exchange of blood or body fluids. The use of condoms gives significant protection, but is not foolproof. Sexual practices to avoid include: anal intercourse; any practice which causes bleeding; oral sex (involving contact between mouth and genitals); sex with male or female prostitutes; sex with any persons who inject themselves with drugs
- not sharing unsterilised needles or syringes between drug users
- women who know or suspect they have HIV not becoming pregnant
- spreading correct information about HIV and AIDS as widely as possible.

How many people have AIDS?

Because HIV infection can remain undetected for many years, no one really knows how many people have the virus. For each case of 'full-blown' AIDS, there may be over 100 infectious carriers. Typically AIDS spreads at an exponential rate, the number of cases doubling in a year: 500 cases become 1 million in 10–11 years. At the end of 1991, WHO estimated that by the year 2000 there would be 30–40 million people with HIV infection, of whom 12–18 million would have AIDS.

Throughout the 1980s the majority of confirmed AIDS sufferers were in the rich world, particularly the USA. WHO figures suggest that by the year 2010 over 90% of HIV infected people will be in developing countries.

One million HIV infections per year are estimated for Africa in the mid-1990s. The annual infection rate in Asia could be in excess of 1 million by the year 2000.

Devastating consequences

On the face of it, even 12–18 million cases of AIDS by the year 2000 does not make it the major killer disease of the late 20th century. *fourteen million children die every year*, mainly from diseases which are preventable; 500 million people are constantly undernourished, leaving them prone to a host of deadly infectious illnesses. It is not difficult to find tragic statistics which match or surpass the horror of AIDS. Does this single condition really warrant the worldwide concern, the scaremonger publicity and the devotion of billions of dollars that the search for a cure devours?

AIDS in perspective
WHO estimates 12–18 million AIDS sufferers by the year 2000 (the number of resulting deaths, and over what time period, is more difficult to predict).

Other epidemics
Bubonic plague (the 'Black Death') killed 17–28 million people – one-third to one-half of Europe's population – between 1347 and 1350.
Influenza killed 22 million in the 1917–18 pandemic.
Smallpox killed 400,000 Europeans at the height of the 19th-century epidemic.

Other causes of death
Diarrhoea kills 5 million children annually.
Malaria kills 2 million people each year.
Ethiopian famine killed 1 million people during 1984–85.
Vietnam war killed 2½ million people between 1960 and 1975.

Source: based on chart from *World Watch*.

Beyond the numbers game, the media outrage at the rising totals of dead and dying, lies the true gravity of AIDS. More than just a new disease, it is a devastating condition which strikes at the heart of any society: its sexually active and economically productive generations. By selecting breadwinners and parents among its victims, AIDS destroys families and reduces the available workforce. Through transmission from mother to unborn child, HIV ensures that future generations will not be spared. The ultimate twist in this tragic story is revealed in WHO's prediction that by the year 2010, 90% of those infected will be in the developing world. In communities already ravaged by poverty and malnutrition emerges a new killer disease; at a time when real progress is being made to save the lives of young children comes an illness which carries off their parents.

A family in Kenya

Tom doesn't have AIDS – yet. But when his blood was tested for HIV the result was positive. For two months he made peace with himself. He read a lot about AIDS, understood how it is transmitted and thought about the likelihood of his developing the full-blown disease. Unlike many of his friends, he is faithful to his wife. He then plucked up courage and told her.

When I talked to Tom, his wife was still in a state of shock. He is 40, she is 36. They have three children, aged eleven, ten and six, and Tom thinks they are too young to be told. He has told his boss, who is sympathetic, but says he won't say anything to his friends or relatives. 'People are very hostile. They think they can get it just by touching you. There's a stigma attached because it's transmitted sexually.'

The most likely explanation for Tom's positive blood test is that the virus was already present in his wife. Over many years she had numerous blood transfusions during a series of miscarriages, and she estimates that she must have 20 pints of alien blood in her body. Moreover, the blood transfusions were carried out in Uganda where the risk of contracting AIDS is greater than in Kenya.

Tom is remarkably philosophical. 'It will not kill so fast. You can adjust and try to go on normally. I think I'm lucky to know before it becomes so debilitating. And we all have to die sometime. The most important thing is to provide for the children. My plan is to work until I feel I'm weak somehow. I believe that you should be good to yourself and to your neighbour and that you can lead a happy life.'

Tom is hopeful that maybe someone will find a cure. 'We're lucky that the rich countries have AIDS too, because they have the money for research. I've read about some guys who found out they had it and committed suicide, but I'll just wait and hope.'

Source: New Internationalist, March 1987.

Whilst the industrialised world predicts a peak in the annual total of AIDS cases during the 1990s, the developing world braces itself for a pandemic that will have a devastating impact well into the next century. In the countries of Central and Eastern Africa, the disease has already left its mark: more than half the population of some villages in Uganda are HIV infected. In the Masaka region alone it is

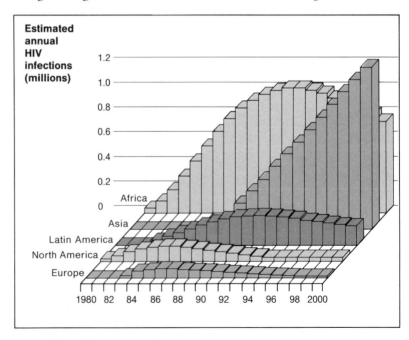

estimated that by 1999 there will be around 250,000 orphans of parents who have died of AIDS. But even more worrying on a global scale is the projected explosion of AIDS victims in Asia, the most populous continent on earth. In Thailand, where the disease was first reported among homosexuals and drug users in 1984, widespread prostitution is thought to have hastened its rapid advance into the heterosexual population. Unless patterns of sexual behaviour change, Thai medical experts predict an HIV-infected population of 4 million by the year 2000, or 1 in 14 Thais.

The longer-term consequences of the spread of AIDS in the developing world can only be guessed at. It is likely that overall adult *life expectancy* will decline, from an estimated 62 years in Africa at the end of the century to 48 years, according to one WHO calculation. *Infant mortality* rates may well rise by up to 50 per thousand births, negating the gains made through immunisation and ORT programmes. Worldwide, some 10 million additional orphans are anticipated. Beyond the individual stories of human suffering and grief will be the enormous social and economic costs created by the sudden transformation of young, healthy adults from societies' producers and carers into consumers of health services who eventually leave their dependants for others to look after.

The 20th-century plague

Manchester's former Chief Constable James Anderton once accused homosexuals with AIDS of 'swirling around in a human cesspit of their own making'. *African Aids 'deadly threat to Britain'*, ran a lead headline in the *Sunday Telegraph*, whilst the British government

A leaflet put out by the Terrence Higgins Trust, a charity which supports AIDS sufferers.

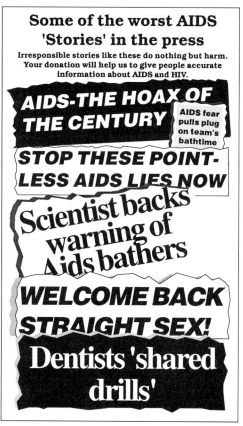

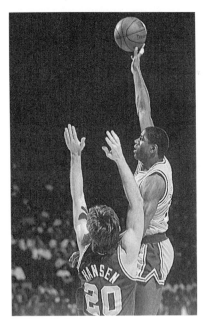

Earvin 'Magic' Johnson, superstar and HIV sufferer.

'There are no "good" or "bad" AIDS patients. For me AIDS is the revelation of the non-acceptance of differences between people.'
Pascale, a student nurse, speaking at a WHO Youth Forum on World AIDS Day, 1988.

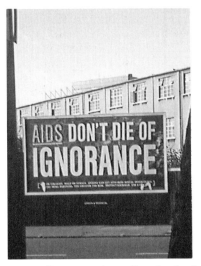

A London street hoarding. Lack of understanding about HIV infection is a major cause of the rapid spread of the disease.

debated in 1986 whether Africans should be submitted to blood tests on entering the UK. Such is the prejudice and misinformation surrounding AIDS that society's reaction to the disease has been likened to the plague mentality which swept Europe in the Middle Ages. The lepers' 20th-century counterparts are homosexuals, Africans and prostitutes. Amongst the human rights abuses reported by AIDS sufferers are denial of medical attention, dismissal from jobs, removal of children from their parents and physical assault.

Despite statistics which showed that, throughout the 1980s, there were more AIDS victims in the USA than in Africa, the myth of 'the African disease' was widespread, leading to discrimination against African residents and visitors in Europe and North America. The other prevailing myth, of AIDS as 'the gay disease', still lingers, resulting not only in further prejudice towards homosexuals but also in a dangerous complacency amongst some heterosexual couples who believe 'it can't happen to us'. The worldwide evidence, on the contrary, indicates that heterosexual intercourse now constitutes the most common form of HIV transmission.

On 7 November 1991, 'Magic' Johnson – the greatest and most popular American basketball star of his generation – announced to a stunned media that he was retiring because he had tested positive for HIV (though he subsequently played in the winning American team at the Barcelona Olympic Games). The same evening Johnson assured America on a late-night talk show that 'I am very far from being a homosexual' and indicated that he had become infected through a sexual encounter with a woman (not his wife whom he had recently married) two months earlier. This admission was significant on two counts: firstly, it distanced Johnson from AIDS sufferers in the gay community whom the media had depicted as being a threat to the health of the nation. Secondly, it alluded to the popular belief that prostitutes are to blame for the spread of AIDS amongst the heterosexual population. In fact, the likelihood of HIV transmission by an infected female to a male is still disputed, but it is certainly much lower than male to female infection.

Fighting ignorance: condoms and cassava leaves

'Don't die of ignorance' was the message of a leaflet distributed to all households in the UK in 1987 in an attempt to counteract the lack of understanding about AIDS amongst the British public. Widespread and reliable information about how to prevent HIV infection remains the principal vehicle for fighting the spread of the disease in both the industrialised and developing worlds. Education programmes, however, constantly run up against the prejudices, taboos and myths that surround AIDS because of its associations with sexual intimacy, an aspect of human behaviour which most people prefer to keep secret. The single most effective preventive measure – the condom – is relatively cheap and widely available; yet a survey in Uganda found that condoms were used by less than 1% of men as such protection was considered 'not manly' and 'Western nonsense'. In addition to the traditional opposition from the Roman Catholic Church to the use of contraceptives, the condom is regarded in many societies as a symbol of promiscuity.

Preventive education in Sierra Leone

'I am Mr Condom . . .' Mr Condom is not the brand name of a contraceptive. He is John G'Bla, a young Freetown artist, whose syncopated song is broadcast on Sierra Leone's national radio. People have certainly heard about AIDS in Freetown, Sierra Leone's capital, but according to a local journalist they consider it a rarity and not much of a threat. And if it becomes one, traditional medicine is there to fight it. One person, for example, thought that eating cassava leaves would serve as a protection. Other false ideas amongst young people include the belief that AIDS is a white man's disease and only homosexuals can catch it.

An illustration from the book on AIDS for primary school students in Sierra Leone, where sexual relations between young people often start at an early age.

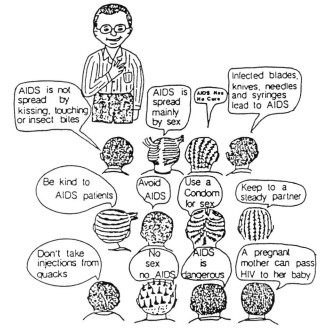

In July 1989 a project on AIDS education was launched throughout the school system in Sierra Leone, using specially written handbooks. The primary school pupil's book, packed with illustrations, begins with the warning 'Take care, AIDS exists in Sierra Leone; AIDS kills . . .' The manual for secondary school pupils presents two characters, a teacher and a nurse, who guide the reader through the chapters. They answer questions put by a pupil and his girlfriend with whom, of course, the readers identify. The pupils also learn how to put on a condom.

However, one of the major objectives of this project is to try to reach those children who do not attend school and who account for over half of the young population. This is attempted by using the informed school children to educate their out-of-school peers. Several activities have accordingly been planned to enable children to pass on the information, such as putting on a puppet or shadow theatre show; producing a radio programme on AIDS using a simple cassette; designing posters on AIDS prevention and composing songs.

And, all the while, the song of Mr Condom can be heard on Freetown radio attracting, it is hoped, many fans among the young people of Sierra Leone.

Source: Unesco Sources no. 17, July/August 1990.

Here I am, a few years on
    it was hard enough explaining
    where Daddy had gone.
She knows there's something
    wrong with me
How can I explain about HIV? . . .
'You don't have these bugs
    darling, so there's no need to
    worry.'
'But you have mummy,' she says
    in a hurry.
'Yes, my lamb, in me these bugs
    grow.'
'When you die mummy, where
    will I go?' . . .
Then we cuddle and I say 'I'm
    here.'
I wish I could take away all her
    fear.
I don't fear dying any more.
Just for a special little girl who's
    only four.

*Written by Ruth, an AIDS
sufferer, for her daughter.*

Source: AVERT (Aids Education
and Research Trust)

*Different worlds, same message.
AIDS information posters
produced by the Kenya Red
Cross Society (left) and a
California Children's Centre
(right).*

Resistance to using condoms is not confined to the developing world. A survey in Britain found that among young women aged 16–24 only 1 in 10 insisted on protected intercourse. The reasons given included embarrassment, religious beliefs, assumptions that their partners were not infected and refusals by men to wear condoms. WHO believes that women have a vital role to play in limiting the spread of AIDS. They are particularly vulnerable to HIV infection from heterosexual intercourse; once infected, the virus can be passed on from mother to unborn child; and, research suggests, mothers bear the burden of responsibility for educating their children about sex and personal relationships. However, women have also lost some of their power to make decisions about sexual relationships which they had gained through the introduction of the pill and other female contraceptive devices. The emergence of HIV leaves women dependent, once more, upon the co-operation and sense of responsibility of their male partners.

Various strategies for imparting information about AIDS have been tried. In the UK, mass advertising campaigns in the 1980s designed to shock young people about the dangers of AIDS have been replaced by gentler, more reasoned appeals to promote the use of condoms. Educating drug addicts has been the focus of a special project in Amsterdam, while in Denmark, a careful study of adolescent lifestyles has led to a programme tailored to meet those needs. Brazil's former football idol, Pele, is being used to get the message across to that country's football-crazy youth; crucial advice is offered from the pulpit in Uganda, a country with a very high rate of church attendance. Free condoms are available from school clinics in New York City to all secondary school students aged 12 and above. In Thailand, elephants have become walking billboards, reminding villagers to *Think Big – Think Condom*; a Bangkok restaurant, called *Cabbages and Condoms*, serves contraceptives with the food, and a senior Thai doctor suggests that primary school children should be encouraged to blow up condoms instead of balloons. These are some of the innovative ways in which health officials and community leaders around the world are attempting to combat the ignorance, myth and prejudice on which the AIDS epidemic flourishes.

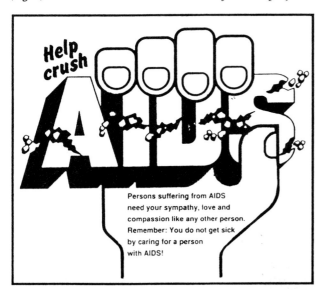

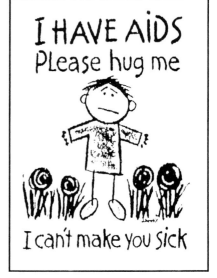

Chasing a cure: the big divide

Whilst the emergence of AIDS constitutes a major headache for health services worldwide, it has presented medical science with an immense challenge: to find a cure before the epidemic decimates the world's population in a way that no other disease has done since the Black Death in Europe. Equally immense will be the profits to the pharmaceutical company which discovers a drug that prevents the development of AIDS or, better still, a vaccine against HIV infection. Some progress has been made, though the virus is particularly complex. The drug AZT, first marketed in 1986, prolongs the lives of some AIDS sufferers by up to three years but does not destroy the virus. An effective HIV vaccine, however, so desperately needed to stem the tide of infection, seems only a remote possibility before the end of the century.

The search for a cure for AIDS shows in sharp and deadly relief the connection between health and wealth. Millions of dollars are spent annually on developing a vaccine, but the strains of the virus being studied are those from the West, not from the developing world. The cost of treating an AIDS patient with AZT is $4000 a year; the total annual health budget of some African countries is less than $5 per person. In fact, AZT is not even obtainable in Africa because, according to its manufacturers, the sophisticated medical infrastructure needed to administer and monitor use of the drug is not available. Diverting some of these countries' scarce resources to treating AIDS would inevitably mean less money for fighting the many other killer diseases. Instead, the typical treatment is necessarily crude: a few days in hospital, some aspirin, then home to die.

Such discrepancies in AIDS treatment are beginning to have a noticeable effect on the course of the disease in rich and poor worlds. From initial infection to the development of full-blown AIDS can take ten years in the West; the average period is less than four years in Africa. Whilst the rate of transmission of HIV from mother to child is 13% in Europe, it is 48% in Kenya. It seems likely that the cumulative effect of malnutrition and other infectious diseases weakens the body's ability to resist the virus or fight off AIDS-related illnesses.

'Expenditure of $1 billion a day on the Gulf War shows that we have the means, if the political will exists, to make policies which ensure that no one is denied the right to be free of AIDS', says Dr Maxine Ankrah of Makerere University in Uganda. 'AIDS calls for a global commitment to an ethical imperative that transcends science. That ethical imperative is that we care.' Perhaps the greatest challenge that AIDS presents to the world's people is not technological but humanitarian: do we care enough to ensure that the most populous and least affluent societies are not destroyed by the '20th-century plague'? Or will AIDS become another entry in the shameful catalogue of 'diseases of poverty' for which a cure exists if you happen to be able to afford it?

'AIDS, more than any other disease, has brought about the realisation that the spread of disease may be more influenced by economic and social dynamics than by biological pathways.'
President Yoweri Musaveni of Uganda, addressing the seventh international conference on AIDS in 1991.

'The AIDS pandemic is exploiting societal weaknesses. The major societal fault lines it proceeds along involve inequality, injustice and discrimination. People are not equal in their ability to protect themselves from HIV because the ability to control personal behaviour is strongly influenced by society.'
Dr Jonathan Mann, Director of the International AIDS Center, Harvard University.

5   The environmental connection

Environment . . . the key to health

AIDS is just one of a number of deadly viruses that have emerged in the second half of the 20th century. Ebola, Lassa fever and Rift Valley fever, whilst much less widespread than AIDS, are all highly infectious and incurable. Interestingly, in each case their emergence coincided with social and environmental changes triggered by development and modernisation. Lassa fever, carried by rodents, first struck in Sierra Leone following the starting up of a new diamond-mining industry; Rift Valley fever has been traced back to the building of the Aswan Dam in Egypt, which created a massive new breeding ground for the disease-carrying mosquitoes; the Ebola virus took hold in a remote part of Zaïre following the opening of a new hospital, where the unavoidable practice of sharing needles spread the disease from one patient to another. There may be thousands more viruses, as yet unknown, lying dormant until further changes to the environment or climate bring them into close contact with the human race.

As we discovered in Chapter 2, the greatest increase in health standards following the industrial revolution came not from vaccines, drugs or surgery but from improving environmental and social conditions: better housing, sanitation and diet. A healthy environment is just as important today. Medical science – and most medical practice – is preoccupied with a *curative* approach to health, finding cures for existing diseases or replacing damaged organs. As important as this approach is, *preventive* medicine is also vital to the long-term and permanent eradication of disease. Central to the preventive approach, which is explored more fully in Part Three, is consideration of the quality of the environment in which we live and work. So long as environmental conditions remain damaging to health, existing diseases will not be overcome and new strains of illness will emerge to baffle the brightest scientific minds.

It could be argued that environmental quality is the single most significant factor in achieving the goal of health for all. In the poorest countries, contaminated water and unsafe sanitation are responsible for more than half of all sickness, whilst industrialisation has wreaked havoc on the environment of the rest of the world in the form of pollution to air, sea and land. Only slowly are we coming to understand the impact of pollution on health but it seems likely that environmental degradation is a contributory cause of most degenerative diseases and a particularly significant factor in the development of many cancers. As well as damaging the earth's life support systems, pollution is destroying life itself. The long-term consequences of our present exploitation of the planet's resources for future generations can only be imagined. This chapter looks at what we know – and suspect – so far.

Water – a matter of life and death

Whilst the industrialised world takes for granted an unlimited supply of chemically treated water, the mere existence of a tap within a short distance from home is a luxury of which many in the rural areas of the poorest countries can only dream. In the rich nations the health debate is about water *quality*: is bottled water better than tap water? Should extra fluoride be added to protect teeth? In two-thirds of the world's households, whose only water source is outside the home, *quantity* is the greater priority. Each person needs a minimum of 5 litres a day for drinking and cooking and 25 more to stay clean; the most a woman (water-haulers are invariably women) can carry in comfort is 15 litres. It is not uncommon for women in parts of Africa to spend five hours a day fetching water for their families.

Water and health

There are four types of water-related disease in the developing world. Each type is transmitted in a different way and therefore requires a particular strategy for prevention.

Means of transmission	Examples of disease	Prevention strategies
1 Water-borne Diseases are carried in water and spread by drinking or washing in contaminated water.	cholera typhoid dysentery	Improve water quality Prevent use of contaminated water

2 Water-washed
Diseases are transmitted from person to person when there is insufficient water for personal and domestic hygiene.
	roundworm
	hookworm
	whipworm
	dysentery
	skin and eye infections
		Increase quantity of
		  water used
		Improve accessibility
		  of water supply
		Improve hygiene

3 Water-based
Diseases are carried by parasitic worms which breed in water snails and then enter the human body through washing or drinking.
	schistosomiasis
	Guinea worm
		Decrease need for
		  contact with infected
		  water
		Improve water quality
		Control snail population

4 Water-related insects
Diseases are transmitted through the bites of insects which breed near water.
	malaria
	river blindness
	sleeping sickness
		Improve management
		  of surface water
		Destroy breeding sites
		  of insects
		Decrease need to visit
		  breeding sites

As *water-washed* diseases are by far the most common, it is more important to increase the *quantity* of water than its *quality* (i.e. it's better to wash your hands in dirty water than not at all). Access to a reliable water supply nearby is critical.

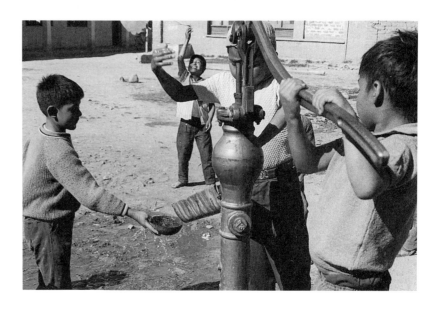

Children in a Bolivian village enjoy pumping water from a recently installed well.

The long walk is over

Mwanaisha Mweropia, a 23 year old mother of six from Mwabungo village in south-eastern Kenya, used to make seven journeys a day to a well some distance away. There was always a line at the well, even at dawn, and the rule was that no one might draw a second bucketful without joining the queue again. Everyone quarrelled and women with large families – which was most of them – were constantly tired. Mwanaisha coughed perpetually and had chronic chest problems.

In 1984 her life changed when the Kenyan Water for Health Organization (KWAHO) installed a handpump in Mwabungo – part of a special project to drill boreholes and install pumps in over a hundred communities. Not only is the handpump much closer to Mwanaisha's home and far less onerous to operate but the water is safe and her cough and chest pains have disappeared. The local KWAHO community worker says that all water-related disease has declined. Before the project, schistosomiasis used to claim around ten lives a year in Mwabungo alone. No one has died from it recently, and the number of diarrhoea cases has dropped by half.

The striking feature of KWAHO's programme is that it was inspired by women, is mostly run by women and has fully involved women in the villages. Each community collects money – a shilling (three pence) a week per family – for repairs and maintenance. To Mwanaisha Mweropia it is a small price to pay for a better, healthier life.

Source: New Internationalist, May 1990.

Every day in the 1980s – the International Drinking Water Supply and Sanitation Decade – about 200,000 people gained a safe supply of drinking water and 80,000 a better means of sanitation. Despite this considerable achievement, population growth over the same period meant that 300 million more people lacked sanitation in 1990 than in 1980. The Decade's goal of 'safe water and sanitation for all by 1990' was never really achievable, despite the co-ordinated efforts of several international organisations. Instead of high-

A decade of progress

The UN International Drinking Water Supply and Sanitation Decade was launched to provide 'water and sanitation for all by 1990'. This ambitious target was never realisable and 300 million more people lacked sanitation in 1990 than in 1980. But in percentage terms there has been some progress, especially with water: 50% of people in rural areas now have an adequate water supply compared with only 30% ten years ago.

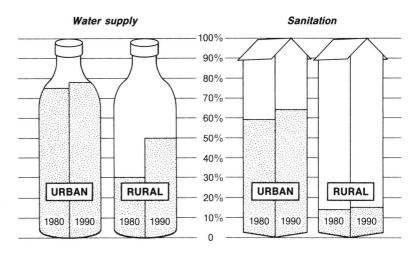

technology water and sewerage treatment systems, which were complex and expensive to maintain and often useless if they broke down as spare parts were unobtainable locally, development agencies now believe that low-cost, simple handpumps and latrines are more appropriate. Aid workers now stress the importance of understanding local conditions and customs before applying foreign standards of health and hygiene.

An illustration from Ants, a Zimbabwean children's comic which publishes important information as well as stories and puzzles.

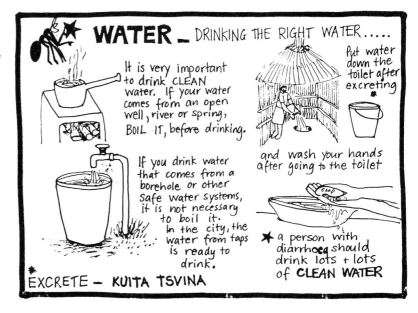

Whilst international attention is rightly focused on supplying safe water and sanitation, water-related disease continues to spread. Malaria remains a very serious environmental health problem, compounded by poor drainage of stagnant waters, ill-conceived irrigation schemes and inappropriate use of pesticides – all of which have contributed to a growing population of mosquitoes and to strengthening their resistance to insecticides. An epidemic of cholera threatens 120 million people in South America, the latest victims of a pandemic which has swept across the world from Indonesia since 1961. Cholera bacteria, found in dirty water and contaminated food, can quickly lead to death from diarrhoea, particularly in young children. Cholera, however, is just one of the many water-related causes of diarrhoeal infection, which kills 5 million children annually. Water, so necessary for life, is also a truly deadly drink.

Air – a chemical cocktail

Whereas water threatens the lives of countless millions in the developing world, the health of those living in industrialised areas is jeopardised by another life-giving force – air. More than one billion people – one-fifth of humanity – live in areas where the air is not fit to breathe, according to UN statistics. The effect on health is frightening. In Athens the number of deaths increases sixfold on heavily polluted days; breathing the air in Bombay is reckoned to be the equivalent of smoking ten cigarettes a day; and the American Lung Association estimates that air pollution costs the US $40 billion annually in health care and lost productivity.

A power station in Delhi, India. Air pollution is a major threat to the health of people living in urban areas.

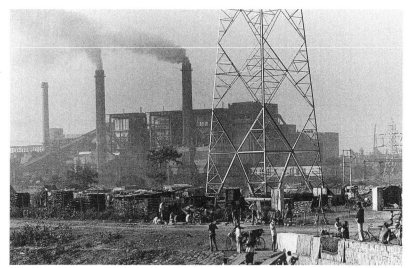

The burning of fossil fuels – predominantly coal – by power stations, factories and in homes was the first air-borne health hazard to be recognised. London's 'great smog' in 1952 claimed 4000 lives from respiratory diseases caused by sulphur dioxide emissions and other pollutants; the ensuing public outcry propelled the passing of the 1956 Clean Air Act and a reduction in domestic coal-burning. Whilst sulphur dioxide pollution has declined in most affluent countries – though Milan, Paris and Madrid still regularly exceed WHO's acceptable limits – it remains a serious threat to health in developing-world cities and in Eastern Europe. Reliance on brown coal, which is cheap and abundant but poor in quality and high in sulphur, has had devastating consequences in the major industrial regions of Czechoslovakia, Poland and the former East Germany. Incidences of respiratory illness and cancer are 30–50% higher in these areas than the national averages, rates of infant mortality and abnormality have risen and life expectancy has declined. Sulphur dioxide is not solely to blame: metals such as lead, zinc, cadmium and mercury – the waste products of heavy industry – have so contaminated the soil and water supplies that they now enter the body through the food chain.

Through enforced pollution control measures and greater energy efficiency, the cleaning up of industry is under way in many countries. At the same time, the battle for clean air is being thwarted by the most prized symbol of Western industrialisation: the car. In the rich world, cars (and other vehicles) are responsible for 75% of all carbon monoxide emissions, 50% of nitrogen oxides and 40% of hydrocarbons. The collective toll of this chemical cocktail includes respiratory infections, cancer and impaired mental and physical development. Ground-level ozone, formed when sunlight causes hydrocarbons to react with nitrogen oxides, is now the major constituent of urban smog, the thick haze which frequently encases cities such as Los Angeles, causing severe respiratory problems and long-term lung damage. The most widely recognised car pollutant, lead, is being substantially reduced by increased use of lead-free petrol, though its harmful effects on children were suspected almost as soon as it was introduced in the 1920s. In the decade following US government regulations on lead in fuel, the average lead level in Americans' blood dropped more than one-third. A study in Mexico City, however, found lead levels in the blood of 7 out of 10 newborn babies to exceed WHO safety standards. 'The implication', says Mexican chemist and environmentalist Manuel Guerra, 'that an entire generation of children will be intellectually stunted is truly staggering.'

'Lean-burn' engines, catalytic converters and alternative fuels will undoubtedly help reduce toxic emissions from cars, but cleaner air may not be achieved until better public transportation, car-pooling schemes and commuting by bicycle reduce the number of cars on

Health effects of pollutants from automobiles

Pollutant	Health effect
Carbon monoxide	Interferes with blood's ability to absorb oxygen impairing perception and thinking, slows reflexes, causes drowsiness, and can cause unconsciousness and death; if inhaled by pregnant women, may threaten growth and mental development of foetus.
Lead	Affects circulatory, reproductive, nervous, and kidney systems; suspected of causing hyperactivity and lowered learning ability in children; hazardous even after exposure ends.
Nitrogen oxides	Can increase susceptibility to viral infections such as influenza. Can also irritate the lungs, and cause bronchitis and pneumonia.
Ozone	Irritates mucous membranes of respiratory system; causes coughing, choking and impaired lung function; reduces resistance to colds and pneumonia; can aggravate chronic heart disease, asthma, bronchitis and emphysema.
Toxic emissions	Suspected of causing cancer, reproductive problems and birth defects. Benzene is a known carcinogen.

[1]Automobiles are a primary source, but not the only source, of these pollutants.
Source: National Clean Air Coalition and the US Environmental Protection Agency. Table taken from *World Watch*.

the road. Meanwhile, car sales continue to rise worldwide and their pollutants contribute to the atmospheric build-up of carbon dioxide and other 'greenhouse gases' that could herald major climatic changes within the next 25–50 years. Higher temperatures and rising sea levels are widely predicted, but the impact of global warming on disease patterns could be equally dramatic. As the climate warms, diseases which flourish in hot, humid weather – such as polio, cholera, dysentery – could increase in formerly temperate regions. Changes in temperature and rainfall may also affect the breeding habits of disease-carrying insects such as mosquitoes and worms, spreading malaria and other tropical diseases into areas such as Europe and Australasia, where people's natural resistance is low. Already being felt are the health consequences of a related global environmental problem, the depletion of ozone in the upper atmosphere. The risk of melanoma, a skin cancer whose rate is growing faster than any other cancer, is now 15 times greater than it was 60 years ago. The health of future generations may suffer not so much from the quality of the air they breathe but more from the long-term damage to the earth's atmosphere inflicted on them by their ancestors.

What is your view of city life in the year 2025? The extract is taken from Veena Hari, 'My Home City', from an unpublished essay reproduced in Children and the Environment, *UNEP/Unicef, 1990.*

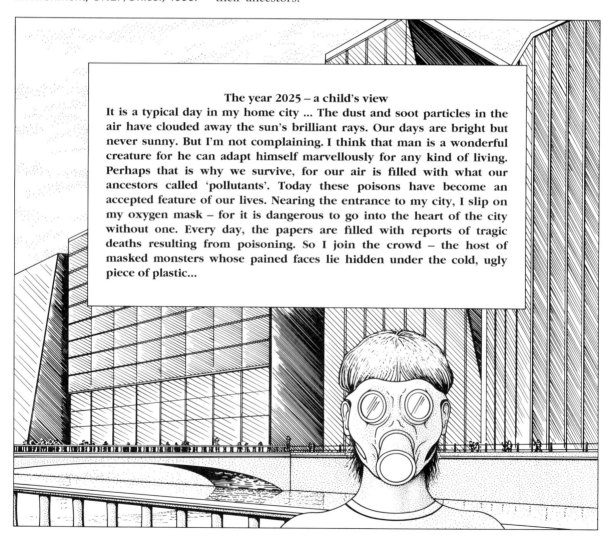

The year 2025 – a child's view

It is a typical day in my home city ... The dust and soot particles in the air have clouded away the sun's brilliant rays. Our days are bright but never sunny. But I'm not complaining. I think that man is a wonderful creature for he can adapt himself marvellously for any kind of living. Perhaps that is why we survive, for our air is filled with what our ancestors called 'pollutants'. Today these poisons have become an accepted feature of our lives. Nearing the entrance to my city, I slip on my oxygen mask – for it is dangerous to go into the heart of the city without one. Every day, the papers are filled with reports of tragic deaths resulting from poisoning. So I join the crowd – the host of masked monsters whose pained faces lie hidden under the cold, ugly piece of plastic...

Toxic waste – the price of progress?

In the mid-1980s, two catastrophic accidents shocked the world and starkly revealed the health risks involved in commonplace industrial processes. During the routine production of a pesticide in 1984, a massive quantity of methyl isocyanide gas was released from the Union Carbide plant in Bhopal, India. Three thousand people died, 20,000 were injured and over half a million Bhopal citizens continue to suffer the effects of serious poisoning, ranging from abortions and stillbirths to respiratory complaints and reduced immunity to infection. Two years later the Chernobyl 4 nuclear reactor, mistakenly regarded as one of the most reliable in the world, exploded and hurled the contents of its radioactive core across Europe. The exact toll of this disaster will never be known but it is now admitted that the thyroid glands of more than 150,000 people were seriously affected by radioactive iodine, that rates of thyroid cancer among people living in the affected areas are 5–10 times

Cancer and the environment

The causes of cancer are much disputed. It is probable that there is a range of contributory factors, some hereditary, some psychological, some to do with environment and lifestyle. The links between cancer and the environment seem especially strong in industrialised societies, where thousands of synthetic chemicals are in regular use.

In the factory

Many industrial processes involve the use of carcinogenic (cancer-causing) substances. Particularly dangerous are asbestos, vinyl chloride (used in making plastics) and benzene. Safety equipment, such as protective masks, should be worn by all workers thought to be at risk.

On the farm

Agriculture is now heavily dependent upon chemical pesticides and herbicides, which act faster than biological forms of pest control. Some, like DDT, are known to be carcinogenic and have been banned in the West. Others, like Paraquat (containing the same active ingredient as the notorious defoliant used in Vietnam), are subject to strict controls. Farm workers are at risk, particularly if working without protection.

At home

Links have been established between lung cancer and people living in houses containing a high quantity of naturally occurring radon gas. Living in a house with a smoker – even if you do not smoke yourself – also increases the risk of lung cancer.

At the table

Pesticide residues on fresh fruit and vegetables may cause cancer – though the quantity needed to be consumed is disputed. More certain is the link between diet and cancer – people who eat a lot of fatty, smoked or salted food are particularly susceptible.

In the neighbourhood

Living or working near a petro-chemical plant or a nuclear power station could be dangerous. So, too, could the proximity of a toxic waste dump. The safe disposal of toxic wastes – the unwanted by-products of industrial processes – is now a major worldwide problem.

Under the sun

A big increase in cases of melanoma, a skin cancer, is linked to greater exposure to harmful ultraviolet rays from the sun due to ozone depletion in the upper atmosphere. Fair-skinned people are particularly at risk, especially if not using sun-block lotions.

higher than would normally be expected, and that leukaemia rates among children are 2–4 times above normal levels. About 200,000 people have been forced to leave their homes in contaminated areas of the Ukraine, Byelorussia and Russia. Radiation from the disaster took just 11 days to reach the east coast of the United States, some 5000 miles away.

It was intentional, rather than accidental, human activity which caused a major environmental disaster in 1991. Military precision during the Gulf War not only killed thousands of civilians directly, it released a stew of contaminants which made breathing hazardous for those who survived. Huge clouds of smoke from the burning oil, blocking out sunlight and turning day into night, were responsible for the persistent sore throats that afflicted virtually everyone in Kuwait. The long-term impact of exposure to such concentrated air pollution is unknown, but a 10% rise in Kuwait's death rate is forecast by WHO. Worldwide, military activity – whether part of actual combat or not – poses one of the greatest threats to environmental health. The military is the single largest producer of hazardous wastes in the USA, generating more than the top five chemical companies combined. 'The most contaminated square mile on earth' is a description of the Rocky Mountain Arsenal near Denver, Colorado, where 125 different chemicals have been dumped during 30 years of nerve-gas and pesticide production. The potential use of such deadly weapons of mass destruction is too horrendous to contemplate.

Pesticide use in agriculture, designed to improve crop yields, is another threat to health that is little understood or publicised. Isolated media stories, such as the withdrawal in 1989 of the apple spray Alar, once links to cancer in children had been confirmed, remind us of the dangers; but overall, some 25% of chemicals sprayed on food are thought to be *carcinogens*. The most immediate victims of the widespread use of chemicals in agriculture are farm workers: an estimated 80,000 die annually from accidental pesticide poisoning and more than half a million people are seriously injured. Workers in the developing world are the most vulnerable, partly due to insufficient knowledge of the hazards but also because multinational pesticide manufacturers continue to sell products – such as DDT and Lindane – which have been banned in many industrialised countries on account of the proven risks to health associated with their use.

Carcinogens are substances which encourage the growth of cancer.

'Unfortunately, because of insecticide sprays, an apple a day no longer keeps us away.'

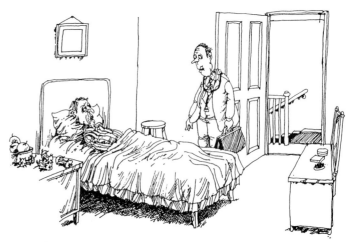

Ironically, the use of DDT – prohibited in over 40 countries – has been sanctioned by the World Health Organisation in Brazil's anti-malaria campaign, funded by the World Bank. DDT is known to be fast-acting and cheaper than any other mosquito-killing pesticide and Brazil faces a major malaria crisis. Evidence from other countries, however, does not augur well for the campaign's success. In addition to its murderous effects on wildlife, widespread application of DDT in India has introduced the chemical into the food chain; the resultant daily dose of pesticide in the average Indian's diet is at a level described by WHO as potentially damaging to the heart, liver, kidneys and brain. And the mosquito may have the last laugh. Because of its phenomenal reproductive capacity – a single female mosquito resistant to DDT can create up to 20 million offspring in two months – a new plague of malaria-carrying insects is likely to evolve, as has occurred in India. Brazil's understandable desire for a quick solution to the world's most pervasive tropical disease could end up causing long-term damage to her environment and to human health. Is this a price worth paying?

More generally, to what extent is environmental degradation – and the inevitable consequences for health – a price worth paying for the products and practices we have come to associate with the modern, consumer-oriented and chemically dependent society? This question raises profound moral and ethical considerations for us all, whether presently healthy or not.

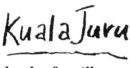

death of a village

Here
intimations of death
hang
heavy in the air
Everywhere
there is the stench
of decay and despair

The river
strangled by
exigencies of
industrialisation
is dying . . .
and nobody cares

The fish
in the river
poisoned by progress's
vomit
are dying . . .
and nobody cares

The birds
that feed on the fish
in the river
poisoned by
progress's excrement
are dying . . .
and nobody cares

And so
a once-proud village
sustained
for centuries
by the richness
of this river
dies . . .
and nobody cares

To that mammon
DEVELOPMENT
our high-priests
sacrifice
our customs
our culture
our traditions
and environment
and nobody cares

We blind mice
We blind mice
see what we've done
see what we've done
we all ran after
Progress's wife
she cut off our heads
with Development's knife
have you ever seen
such fools in your life
as we blind mice?

Cecil Rajendra (a Malaysian poet)

Source: Hope for the Earth? (Harvest 1988 leaflet), Christian Aid.

6   The People versus HealthCare plc

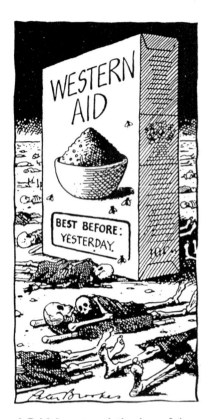

A British cartoonist's view of the effectiveness of Western development aid. In 1990, only four industrialised countries – Norway, The Netherlands, Denmark and Sweden – were giving the amount of aid agreed by UN member states. Only about 5% of all aid given is devoted to health care; only 2% is spent on primary health care and primary education combined, though these are two of the most needed services in poor countries.

In Part Two so far we have seen how complex health issues are, particularly when viewed on a global scale. There are no easy solutions because health is inevitably tied up with political, economic, social, cultural and environmental considerations. Those who make decisions – the health care professionals – are often faced with difficult choices and moral dilemmas. Which diseases should be given priority for research purposes? Whose lives should be saved whilst others are left to die? How should advice be given, or laws passed, which challenge cherished beliefs or reduce company profits? Of course, the consumers of health care – ordinary people – do not necessarily agree with the decisions that have been made on their behalf. As we near the end of the 20th century, health care is not only a major concern of all people but one of the fastest-growing worldwide industries. It is not surprising, perhaps, that individual needs and the motives of profit-making companies are not always in harmony; and that the priorities and practices of governments and international organisations, however well-intentioned, only serve to add to the confused picture.

This chapter tries to summarise some major controversies surrounding health care in a simplified form. Some issues are controversial because they are to do with political or economic choices, others because they involve moral or ethical judgments. The setting is a trial in an imaginary World Court. The case to be heard concerns the following allegation: *that the health of ordinary people does not benefit sufficiently from the health care industry.* Speaking for the Prosecution are representatives – from rich and poor nations and various social and cultural groups – of *The People*. Representing the Defence are officials from *HealthCare plc*, a worldwide conglomerate of health industries, government health departments and international organisations. The Judge? Well ... you can be the Judge! When you have read and reflected on the arguments presented you should come to a decision. Would you find HealthCare plc *guilty* or *not guilty* of the charge? In passing judgment you might also want to make some recommendations for future action by either or both parties.

The economic argument

The People

> *The case, put very simply, is this: not enough money is being spent on health care, particularly in the developing world. It has been estimated that a programme to prevent the great majority of the 100 million child deaths predicted for the 1990s would cost an additional $2.5 billion per year. 'Two and a half billion dollars is a substantial sum,' says Unicef's annual report,* The State of the World's Children 1990. *'It is 2% of the poor world's own arms*

spending. It is the approximate cost of five Stealth bombers. It is as much as the world as a whole spends on the military every day.' Some 90 countries spent more public funds on their military than on health care during the 1980s. To put it crudely, keeping the world's military forces going is killing millions of children.

Secondly, money that is spend on health care does not benefit all people equally. The nations that spend most on health are mainly in the industrialised world, where fewer people suffer from disease and malnutrition. Only 5% of global expenditure on health research is devoted to the health problems of developing countries, where 80% of the world's people live. And thirdly, the proportion of development aid from Western industrialised nations allocated to health declined by one-third during the 1980s. In short, the health of the majority of the world's people is not seen as a priority.

HealthCare plc

The health care industry cannot be blamed for governments' decisions about military spending. However, in recent years we have seen the beginning of a decline in this expenditure in many countries. The end of the Cold War has led to a reduction in military forces and weapons in the industrialised world; many African and Latin American nations are importing fewer arms. The immediate impact, of course, is the loss of jobs – an estimated half a million in the European arms industry alone. Happily, the health care industries are among the fastest growing in the Western world, accounting for 12% of total GDP in the USA. Spending on health in the developing world, however, is still much lower than it should be because of one overriding problem: debt. In the least developed countries, debt-servicing – paying interest on loans – takes up more money than health and education combined. 'Must we starve our children to pay our debts?' asked Tanzania's former President Julius Nyerere. Until the money-lenders – rich governments, the World Bank and the International Monetary Fund – agree to write off debts owed by the world's poorest people, the answer will be 'Yes'.

GDP: Gross Domestic Product, the annual total of revenue generated within a country's borders.

The tragic irony of the debt problem, as seen by an American cartoonist. In 1992, the developing world owed about $1300 billion to the governments and banks of the industrialised nations. Repayments on these loans amount to some $150 billion a year – roughly three times as much as the developing world receives in aid. The poorest countries simply cannot afford to meet their repayments, thereby increasing their debts and crippling their chances of future economic recovery.

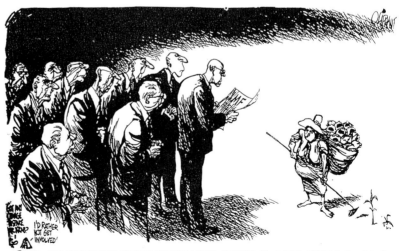

'...SO YOU SEE, THE ENTIRE FUTURE OF THE INTERNATIONAL FINANCIAL SYSTEM HINGES ON YOUR CAPACITY FOR QUICK RECOVERY AND VAST ECONOMIC GROWTH.'

The advancement of medical knowledge tends to occur in the industrialised world because that's where the research money and personnel are, but once a breakthrough happens it can benefit everyone. After all, it was in the rich world that the importance of clean water and sanitation was first demonstrated. The allocation of aid from rich to poor countries is not in our hands: aid is rarely given free of conditions, which often insist on the money being spent on certain products – usually to be purchased from the donor country. And let's not forget that only four rich countries have reached the UN target for development aid of 0.7% of GNP. Rich world governments are deciding that they cannot afford to give more to the poorer nations – and these governments are all democratically elected by The People!

The technological argument

The People

> *Our case is summarised very well by Dr Halfdan Mahler, formerly Director General of WHO: 'Thirty years ago modern health technology had just awakened and was full of promise. Since then, its expansion has surpassed all dreams, only to become a nightmare. For it has become over-sophisticated and over-costly. It is dictating our health policies unwisely; and what is useful is being applied to too few.' Dr David Morley of the London Institute for Child Health explains the situation by means of the 'three-quarters rule': three-quarters of spending on health care in developing countries is for urban-based facilities and staff, yet three-quarters of the population live in rural areas; three-quarters of all deaths in these countries can be prevented by relatively simple and low-cost measures, but three-quarters of health budgets go on high-cost curative care.*
>
> *People are not killed by germs, but by the conditions that allow a disease to overwhelm them. How else can you explain the fact that measles is nearly 250 times more likely to kill someone in Ecuador than in the USA? The money spent on research in a Western laboratory for a measles vaccine would have been spent much more wisely on providing clean water, sanitation and better nutrition in the places where the disease is a killer. In the industrialised world a*

High-tech drugs can help fight disease, but they are expensive to produce.

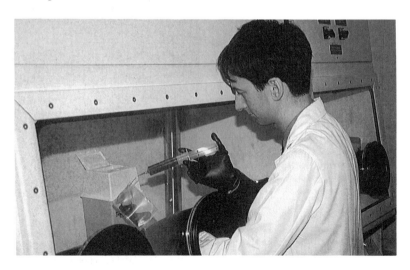

vast proportion of health expenditure is devoted to high-tech 'cures' – organ transplants, anti-cancer drugs, AIDS vaccines – rather than to understanding and changing the conditions which cause these diseases. The health care industry is being ruled by an unquenchable thirst for new technology, rather than by the needs of ordinary people. 'High-tech' – a reliance on technology alone – should be replaced by 'high-touch' – a greater dependence upon the caring and self-healing capacities of human beings.

HealthCare plc

Scientific research is needed to help combat disease. Sir Alexander Fleming's discovery of penicillin has saved countless millions of lives; the smallpox vaccine has eradicated a disease which once killed 2 million people a year. Biotechnology has helped us to understand the significance of genes and how hereditary information is carried by the chemical DNA – knowledge which has a vast range of potential benefits, from preventing genetic disorders (which affect about 2% of live births) to finding an anti-malarial vaccine and eradicating malnutrition through improving crop yields. Although we know that social and environmental factors contribute to cancer, we don't know exactly how or why the disease affects certain people and not others. As more than half of all cancer cases now occur in the developing world, this research is of worldwide importance. And it's probably easier to develop an AIDS vaccine than to change the sexual habits of the hundreds of millions of people who are at risk.

An accepted measure of development and social progress is access to sophisticated health care. Christiaan Barnard, the first heart transplant surgeon, twice lectured in the massive football stadium in Rio de Janeiro to a capacity audience, most of whom were Brazilian

Poster campaigns, like this one in Owo, Nigeria, have encouraged parents to have their children immunised.

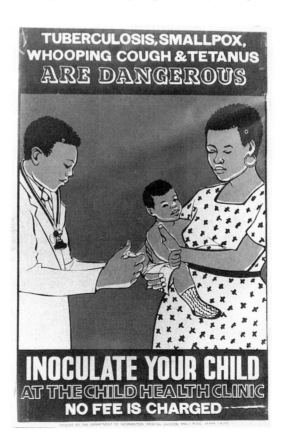

53

peasants who had little hope of ever benefiting from such medical technology. If medicine can prolong lives, or improve their quality, people – quite naturally – want it. But don't forget the highly successful low-cost campaigns that we have undertaken recently in the developing world: the immunisation and oral rehydration therapy programmes and the low-tech achievements of the International Drinking Water Supply and Sanitation Decade.

The moral argument

The People

Some of those people listening to Dr Christiaan Barnard may have had children who have since been caught up in the grim trade of illegal adoptions, in which Brazilian babies are allegedly sold and then killed in Europe so that their organs can be used for transplants. Is this what is meant by progress – health for the wealthy, at any price? Organ transplants are good examples of high-tech medicine for the privileged few: the greater the spending on such expensive surgery, the less money can be devoted to other, less 'glamorous', health problems and preventive health care. The moral principle guiding the allocation of limited resources, in any country, should be the greatest good for the greatest number – that may be different from achieving the best for each individual patient.

In the rich world we are obsessed with prolonging life: 60% of health expenditure in the USA is devoted to people in their last year of life. Their quality of life is not considered. In fact, those who would prefer to die are prevented from doing so by drugs and by laws forbidding euthanasia. This is an extravagant waste of resources. As Michael Wilson, author of Health is for People *has argued, 'only when we are prepared to let some people die will we be free to make more humane decisions in the distribution of resources'. A similar concern for saving life, irrespective of its quality, can be found in the poorer nations, where successful immunisation and ORT programmes are simply condemning more children to a life of poverty and malnutrition. Unless the basic human needs – clean water, food, shelter, education – are satisfied as well, medicine just raises false hopes.*

Keeping a patient alive in an intensive care unit. Is this a wise use of health resources?

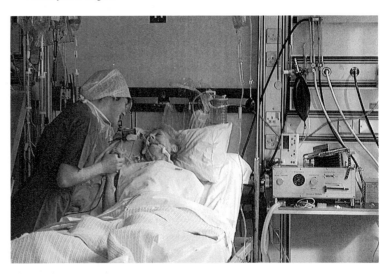

HealthCare plc

Surely you're not suggesting that we should let people die, even though we have the means to keep them alive? I don't think many people would feel happy about health care professionals playing at God, deciding who should live and who shouldn't. Where's the morality in that? As the strong anti-abortion lobby constantly reminds us, life is sacred and our primary responsibility is to preserve it if at all possible. The doctrine of 'the greatest good for the greatest number' is all very well, but what is a doctor or health worker supposed to do when faced with a patient who obviously needs treatment? Does she turn him away just because the treatment is expensive? No, her job is to look after the needs of each patient as best she can.

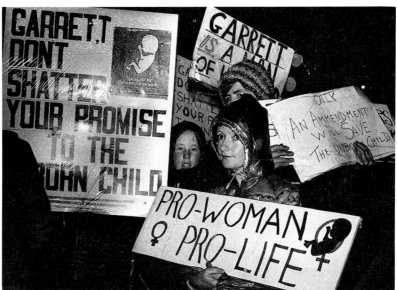

Anti-abortion demonstrators in Ireland campaigning for the unborn child's 'right to life'.

The diseases of modern society are complex, as AIDS and other deadly viruses demonstrate, and therefore costly to overcome. But if we didn't spend money on research and treatment, we wouldn't make any progress towards curing or eradicating them. Future generations wouldn't thank us for that! Medicine has played a crucial role in improving quality of life, particularly for the elderly whose suffering from various diseases and disabilities can be reduced through drugs and surgery. Can it be morally right to let our old people die or live in pain unnecessarily? Should we stop immunising children in the developing world against infectious diseases simply because we don't think their future lives will have sufficient quality? Who can or should judge the quality of someone else's life?

The commercial argument

The People

Our final point is that, despite all their glossy advertising about caring for people, the health care industry views health as a product to be bought. In fact, the advertisements reveal their true concern: without this drug or that dietary plan, this vitamin or that brand of

Antibiotics are drugs, originally derived from moulds and fungi, which either kill bacteria or prevent them from multiplying. *Penicillin* is a common example.

A cartoon from Health Alert, an information network in the Philippines, showing how they believe baby milk companies are discouraging mothers from breastfeeding. Doctors agree that breast milk is the best food for all babies under six months.

babymilk, you can't be healthy. Where are the advertisements encouraging better education for women or cleaner air in cities? Both of these commodities would have a far more beneficial impact on personal health than swallowing pills. Drugs are promoted as the answer to all our problems, yet many prescriptions are unnecessary and some are downright harmful. An estimated 22% of antibiotics used in hospitals are prescribed unnecessarily; these so-called 'miracle-cures' are still found in nearly half of all preparations for treating diarrhoea, despite WHO's advice that they are not suitable. Vitamins are promoted worldwide as essential food supplements, though a nutritionally balanced diet contains an adequate supply of all vitamins, is more enjoyable and a lot cheaper.

In the rich world our bodies are treated as disposable playthings. Surgical fashions come and go with no medical justification – 30 years ago, children's tonsils and appendixes were whipped out, now that's deemed unnecessary. Women are particularly susceptible to the notion of 'doctor knows best'. In childbirth, the most natural of human events, medicine increasingly intervenes through inappropriate surgery – a quarter of all American babies are delivered by Caesarian section – and unwanted drugs, prescribed by 'specialists' of whom most are men. And throughout the developing world, women's bodies are portrayed as no longer proficient at another natural and health-giving function – breastfeeding. Despite persistent condemnation from WHO and Unicef, food and drug companies continue to reap huge profits from the sale of artificial breast milk substitutes which have been proven to contribute substantially to the number of child deaths from diarrhoea. This is

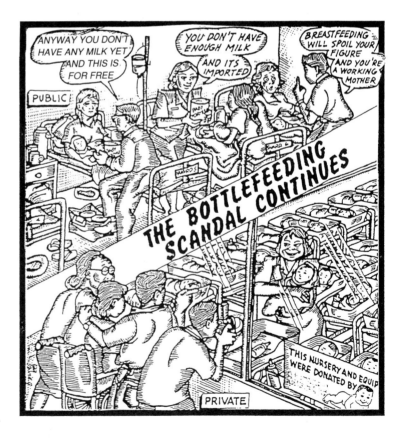

the commercial side of health care at its most cynical: persuading poor and illiterate women that they are incompetent mothers unless they purchase an expensive and potentially lethal substitute for their own milk. That's greed, not care.

HealthCare plc

What a catalogue of accusations! Surely the health care industry cannot be held responsible for the state of the environment and literacy rates – those are the concerns of others. You make an important point, though, that people need to be given more responsibility for their own health. Many health products, such as drugs and vitamins, allow people to control pain or compensate for inadequacies in their diet and lifestyle – so that they don't have to suffer. As people become wealthier and live longer, they want these handy aids. In the poorest countries, too, drugs can provide some relief and hope for people living in despair and poverty.

But personal responsibility can only go so far: medical expertise is needed as well. When women were left to their own devices in childbirth, the infant and maternal mortality rates were higher. Why should they have to suffer in bringing children into the world when medicine can make giving birth less painful and safer? And don't forget it is lack of personal responsibility that creates many health problems – smoking, over-eating and alcohol abuse are common examples. In our high-stress society, people cannot be expected to manage their health by themselves. As for the baby milk argument, that's been debated many times before. Some mothers find it just too difficult or too painful to breastfeed their babies; women who are undernourished themselves appreciate having a milk substitute that will give their babies a good start to life. In any case, it's well known that most companies are now promoting 'follow-up' milks, for babies of over six months, which do not contravene WHO regulations . . .

What's wrong with bottle-feeding? Satisfied infants sleep peacefully in a day-centre in Ecuador.

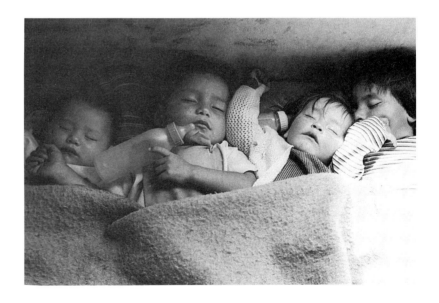

7   Primary health care: putting people first

The little Somali girl lay on a bundle of rags under a fierce late morning sun outside her nomad family's aqal *(hut). Her breathing was slightly laboured, coming out in long drawn-out rasps. Yonis Sheik Ahmed crouched beside the girl, felt her pulse and took her temperature. 'Little pneumonia, not much serious', Yonis whispered. He dug into his black bag and gave a bottle of an antibiotic syrup to the mother, carefully explaining the dosage. He asked her to take the child inside, out of the heat.*

Yonis slung his bag over his shoulder, shook hands and broke into a brisk walk. The next call was a cluster of aqals *nestling on a mountainside opposite, a good hour's walk away via a boulder-strewn goat and donkey track . . .*

Yonis is not a doctor. Before his four months' medical training he had received no formal education. Yet, like many thousands of other *community health workers* all over the developing world, Yonis is playing a significant part in a system of health care that is saving millions of lives and improving health standards in countless communities. The system, known as *primary health care*, emerged in 1978 from a key conference organised by WHO and Unicef in Alma-Ata, in the former Soviet Republic of Kazakhstan. Drawing heavily on the experience of the 'barefoot doctor' movement pioneered by Chairman Mao in China, the Alma-Ata Declaration states that the 'people have the right and duty to participate individually and collectively in the planning and implementation of their health care'. The thinking behind primary health care is simple: given the right information and access to sufficient food, safe water and basic medicines, the principal agents of better health are ordinary people, their families and communities; and that the person best equipped to provide the necessary drugs and knowledge is someone chosen from within the local community.

The essential components of primary health care are those which have featured many times before in this book:
- ensuring an adequate food supply and a balanced diet
- ensuring an adequate supply of safe water and basic sanitation
- promoting education about disease and its prevention
- promoting family planning and contraceptive use
- providing special care for mothers and children
- immunising children against the major infectious diseases
- treating locally common diseases and injuries
- making essential drugs available to everyone.

As this list indicates, the emphasis is on disease prevention. The provision of appropriate food, water and sanitation are the foundations of primary health care. Without them, nothing can be built. But medical expertise is not scorned: the specialist knowledge and equipment found in hospitals is still necessary for treating more serious illness. It is an approach to health care which is relevant to rich and poor countries alike, though it has become associated more with the developing world. Chapter 8 looks at a comparable movement in the industrialised world.

The simplicity of the primary health care ideal should not mask its radical nature. The core of its message is that no one need rely on advanced medical expertise or technology for basic health: and that health care must be available to all, irrespective of wealth, class or creed. 'In virtually all countries,' says Halfdan Mahler, 'primary health care implies a very fundamental social revolution ... I believe that health is a marvellous instrument for giving leverage to people'. Through giving knowledge, responsibility and resources to ordinary people, primary health care promotes social justice as well as health.

Primary health care requires a fundamental change in attitudes, as this illustration from a community health workers' instructors' handbook indicates.

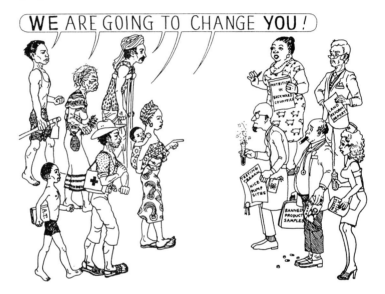

Community health workers

Where There is No Doctor is the title of a best-selling health manual for community health workers. In the industrialised world there is approximately one doctor for every 600 people, whilst the average is close to one doctor for every 17,000 people in the least developed nations. As the majority of people in poorer countries live in rural areas without ready access to fully trained medical personnel, the community health worker plays a pivotal role in the primary health care system. It is much more cost-effective to train a community health worker, at around $500, who will remain in the locality than a doctor, costing at least $60,000, who will work from a distant hospital.

> *Yonis is one of two community health workers in Ruqi, a picturesque village deep inside Somalia's mountainous region of Boroma. Some years ago Ruqi's elders chose Yonis, along with goat herder Mohammud Hajaden, to attend four months' training in*

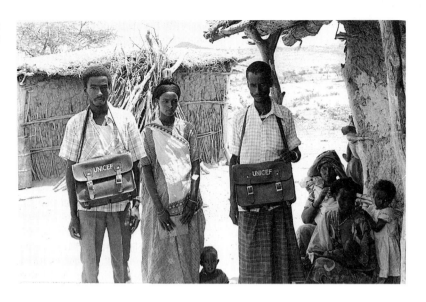

Community health workers Yonis Ahmed and Mohammud Hajaden visiting a homestead in Ruqi, a village in the Baroma region of Somalia.

basic health care run by Unicef and the Somali Ministry of Health in the regional capital. Monitoring the health of some 4000 inhabitants of Ruqi and surrounding nomads' camp sites has been their responsibility ever since. And they're doing a great job, according to the elders. Fewer children fell sick or died, and mothers' health began to improve markedly, within months of Yonis and Mohammud starting their rounds, they say. Each of the pair covers about 20 kilometres on foot every day; the rugged mountain terrain precludes even the use of bicycles. Theirs is a six-day working week and they are on call for seven.

The villagers, mainly shepherds and farmers, have been so happy with the work of their two 'doctors' that they have recently presented 50 goats and sheep to each of them. For two years the community had been unable to raise the monthly wages of 600 Somali Shillings (£5) for the two workers so the elders decided that every household should donate one animal.

'Fantastic', enthused Yonis, who shares a compound with an older sister atop a hill overlooking the village. A goat is twice the monthly wage of a Somali labourer.

Source: Children First!, Unicef UK, Spring 1987.

Not all community health workers operate in the same way: some are full-time, some part-time; some are paid by the community, others by the government. But all of them need to understand the health problems of the community and be able, after a few months' training, to diagnose and treat common illnesses, give vaccinations, advise parents on child care and contraception and recognise when specialist help is required. Perhaps even more important, though, is the task of helping people learn how to meet their own health needs more effectively.

It has been recognised that older children can be successful health workers, particularly in large families where young children are often looked after by their elder siblings. Through *CHILD-to-child*, an international programme started in 1979 by Dr David Morley, children of school age are taught practical information and skills so that they can attend to the health concerns of younger brothers and sisters. Enlisting the enthusiastic help of children not only ensures additional health care for the family but also prepares young people for responsible parenthood.

Focus on women

Another programme which fits the primary health care mould is the *Safe Motherhood Initiative*, launched by WHO in 1987. Recognising that *maternal mortality* is the leading cause of death amongst women in developing countries, the Initiative 'places special emphasis on the need for better and more widely available maternal health services, the extension of family planning education and services, and effective measures aimed at improving the status of women'. It has long been accepted that primary health care should focus particularly on women, partly because they are the traditional child carers and guardians of family health and also because discrimination against girls and women is a major cause of ill-health. In many societies it is customary for girls to work longer hours than boys in the home, but to receive less food, less preventive care and less education than their brothers. Such treatment often contributes to poor health in later life and increases the risks associated with pregnancy and childbirth. In addition, traditional and health-threatening practices such as *genital mutilation* and childhood marriage for girls are widespread in parts of the developing world.

In tackling discrimination and denial of women's rights, primary health care programmes inevitably challenge male-dominated customs and beliefs. Enabling women to exercise more control over

Maternal mortality: death amongst women resulting from complications during pregnancy and/or childbirth.

Genital mutilation, sometimes called *female circumcision:* this practice usually involves the removal of a girl's clitoris together with all or part of the labia minora and majora. It is often performed on young girls by older women in unhygienic conditions, without anaesthetic, causing shock, haemorrhage and infection. Long-term problems include painful menstruation, prolonged and difficult labour and severe psychological and sexual distress. Genital mutilation is a contributory factor in a majority of maternal deaths in Africa, where an estimated 80 million women are affected. Reasons given for the practice include ensuring a girl's virginity until marriage and the 'purification' of female genitals which are considered unclean in some cultures.

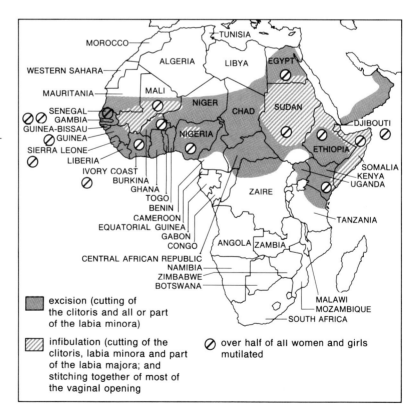

Countries in which genital mutilation of women and girls is widely practised.
Africa and the Middle East, early 1980s.

their own lives is a sensitive issue in most societies, particularly in connection with sexual behaviour and reproduction. It has been shown that family planning can help reduce the number of maternal deaths through preventing unwanted pregnancies, abortions and births to women at high risk. But the pressure on women in the poorest countries to bear many children is considerable, mainly because large families are seen as necessary insurance against the high child mortality rate. An important function of primary health care is to convince women – and their partners – that having fewer children, and adequately spacing their births, actually promotes lower child mortality and increased family health. Evidence from many countries indicates that a decline in population growth follows a decline in levels of poverty: once it can be seen that most babies survive until adulthood, parents are happy to have fewer children. The promotion of family planning and contraception are significant elements of primary health care but their messages are unlikely to be heard unless linked to a much broader programme aimed at the eradication of poverty.

Family planning and contraception are sensitive issues in many communities.

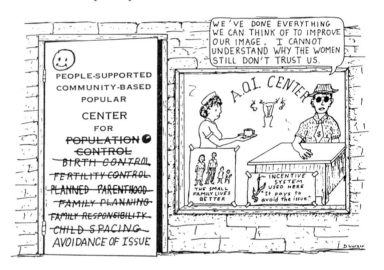

Education: essential for health

For many decades, primary education for all children has been regarded as an essential goal of any country wishing to attain high levels of economic and social development. In Ecuador, Ghana, Kenya and Zimbabwe around one-quarter of total government expenditure is allocated to education, a proportion ten times greater than that found in Canada, Germany, the UK and the USA. Recent statistics have revealed how education and health – the twin pillars on which development has been built – are crucially linked, particularly in respect of the education of girls. According to Unicef, 'education is strongly associated with higher levels of child health and nutrition and lower levels of fertility and infant mortality. On average, every additional year a mother spends at school is associated with a fall in the infant mortality rate of approximately 9 per 1000.'

The present picture, however, is not encouraging. Of the 100 million 6–11 year olds who still do not attend school, 60% are girls, and the drop-out rate for school attenders is far higher amongst girls

'If you educate a man, you educate an individual. If you educate a woman, you educate the whole family.'
Mahatma Gandhi

62

Education and training

Women have made big steps forward since 1970 – but huge gaps persist. Many girls and women still do not receive equal access to education and training.

Literacy
* The number of illiterate people in the world is rising due to population growth. But female illiteracy has risen fastest, from 543 million women in 1970 to 597 million in 1985. Male illiteracy rose from 348 million to 352 million.
* Three-quarters of women aged 25 and over are still illiterate in much of Africa and Asia.

Schooling
* Girls have caught up with boys in some parts of the world, but still lag behind in others.

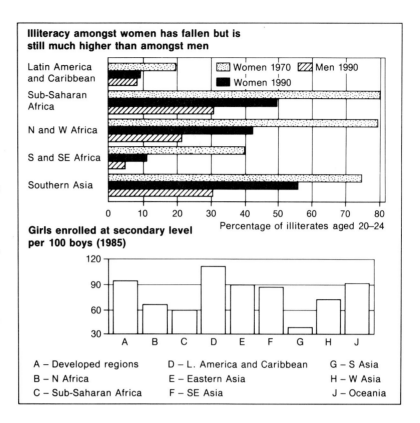

Illiteracy amongst women has fallen but is still much higher than amongst men

Latin America and Caribbean / Sub-Saharan Africa / N and W Africa / S and SE Africa / Southern Asia

Women 1970 / Men 1990 / Women 1990

Percentage of illiterates aged 20–24

Girls enrolled at secondary level per 100 boys (1985)

A – Developed regions   D – L. America and Caribbean   G – S Asia
B – N Africa   E – Eastern Asia   H – W Asia
C – Sub-Saharan Africa   F – SE Asia   J – Oceania

Unesco: the United Nations Educational, Scientific and Cultural Organisation.

than boys. One-third of children enrolled in primary schools in the developing world drop out before completing four grades, the minimum considered necessary for achieving basic literacy. One in four adults in the world – nearly one billion people, of whom two-thirds are women – cannot read or write. Overall, expenditure on primary education declined during the 1980s in more than half of the developing countries and the number of children enrolled in school fell. The reasons for this trend are various, but the burden of debt repayment to the industrialised world is cited as a principal factor by Frederico Mayor, the Director General of Unesco. Heavily-indebted governments cannot afford to expand their education services to keep pace with the increase in their populations.

Although the general picture is gloomy, significant and exciting educational programmes are taking place in some countries. Within the first ten years of independence, the number of Zimbabwean children enrolled in primary schools rose from under 50% to 100%, with three-quarters completing the seven-year course. New classrooms and schools were built, thousands of new teachers were trained and the old British curriculum was gradually phased out in favour of one more appropriate to Zimbabwe's needs. A 20-year literacy campaign in Myanmar (Burma), involving nearly half a million volunteers, has enabled 2 million adults to read and write. Organised by village literacy committees and supported by famous singers, film stars and writers, the campaign receives constant media coverage and appeals to local pride; 'People's Victory' parties are held when a village is declared literate. Another successful low-cost scheme is being pioneered by the Bangladesh Rural Advancement Committee (BRAC). The BRAC programme demonstrates that children can be given a basic education for approximately $15 per year by employing educated community members as teachers and enlisting parents' help in putting up simple classrooms. BRAC schools cater particularly for children of the poorest families and priority is given to girls.

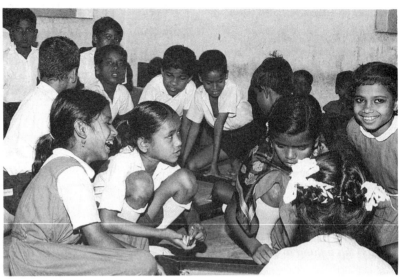

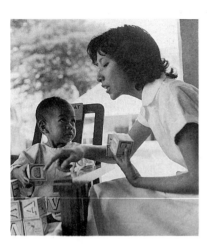

(Above) Education from an early age is important for future health.

At the 1990 World Conference on Education for All in Jomtien, Thailand, sponsored by three UN agencies and the World Bank, three goals for education were set for the 1990s: first, bringing literacy, numeracy and essential life-skills to the great majority of children; second, reducing the adult illiteracy rate to half of its 1990 level; third, ending the great disparity in educational provision between boys and girls. At about the same time an important health-education booklet was published, the outcome of a partnership between the world's leading medical and children's organisations. *Facts for Life* condenses vital knowledge about child and family health into 55 'messages', using simple, non-technical language. The booklet, published in over 80 languages, is aimed at communicators of all kinds – teachers, politicians, religious and business leaders as well as health workers – and urges them to spreads its contents as widely as possible, to men as well as women. 'The greatest communications challenge of all', the booklet suggests, 'is of communicating the idea that the time has come, in all countries, for men to share more fully in that most difficult and important of all tasks – protecting the lives and the health and the growth of their children.'

Progress in primary health care

There are several notable examples of the success of primary health care in enhancing the lives of ordinary people in relatively poor countries. Botswana, whose GNP per capita figure is one-tenth of that in the UK, halved its child mortality rate between 1960 and 1990 and has almost reached its target of immunising 80% of children against major infectious diseases. Community health workers have brought medical assistance within reach of most villagers; nearly 90% of children now attend primary school. A

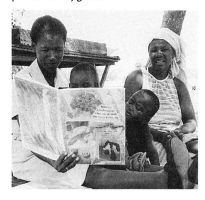

A community health worker in Botswana makes a home visit to explain the importance of personal hygiene.

comprehensive food distribution programme and a malnutrition surveillance scheme have ensured that, even in times of severe drought, no one has died of starvation. In Costa Rica, where the proportion of government spending on health is one of the highest in the world, the infant mortality rate was reduced from 61 to 19 deaths per 1000 births in just ten years through a programme which included all the essential primary health care features. Since abolishing its armed forces in 1948, Costa Rica has maintained remarkable social welfare and education programmes that have contributed to a life expectancy which now exceeds that enjoyed by people in some industrialised nations. The state of Kerala in India provides a shining example of how regional policies aimed at reducing poverty and promoting social equity can raise health standards to a level way above the rest of the country. The infant mortality rate in Kerala is under half the national average, the literacy rate is nearly twice the national average and the birth rate is falling much faster than in the rest of India.

Primary health care, with its emphasis on social justice, is not without its opponents. In the first four years of the Sandinista government in Nicaragua, following the revolution in 1979, 50% of the national budget was devoted to education and health. 'People's Health Councils' were established to co-ordinate nationwide campaigns to eradicate infectious diseases and establish primary health care as a basic human right. From 1983, however, health centres became prime targets of the US-backed military forces known as Contras, and many health workers were kidnapped and executed. As a consequence, immunisation programmes were disrupted, attendance at health centres in the war zones declined, and the number of measles and malaria cases increased. Recent figures indicate that the infant mortality rate rose in the late 1980s, having been cut by half in under ten years. A similar story can be told in Mozambique, which now has the highest child mortality rate in the world. The gains in public health made since independence from Portugal in 1975 have been largely reversed by the attempts of the South African-backed Renamo forces to destabilise the Frelimo government for nearly ten years. Health centres and schools were frequent targets: over 700 health units and more than 2000 primary schools were destroyed in rural areas. An acute shortage of food has added to the health problems of this desperately poor country.

Opposition of a different kind has come from within the medical profession itself. Many doctors, highly qualified in curative medicine and respected people in their own societies, have been sceptical about the effectiveness of a system which emphasises preventive health care and relies on the skills of minimally trained personnel. Some governments, too, have baulked at devoting a large proportion of their health budget to such a low-profile scheme, preferring to spend lavishly on new hospitals and high-tech equipment. As a result, primary health care is regarded by some as a separate, low-cost service for the poor rather than the first tier of a comprehensive health system which caters for the needs of all people. As Halfdan Mahler – eminent doctor, TB specialist and development expert – has put it: 'we have to swing health away from the paternalistic medical wisdom that leads to doling things out and creating dependence. Our greatest difficulty is having the energy, the imagination and the faith to support people when they say "this is what we want".'

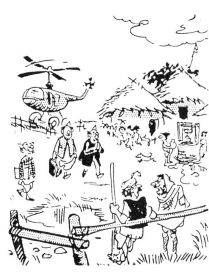

Of course, we have progressed a great deal, first they were coming by bullock cart, then by jeep – and now this!

An Indian cartoonist's view of the role of development experts.

8 Alternative medicine: treating whole people

Traditional medicine

A consultation with the doctor in the 17th century would have entailed much more than a two-minute chat and a scribbled prescription. Questions about your emotional state, your living conditions and the strength of your faith would have featured just as prominently as discussion of your physical symptoms. The doctor would have regarded your state of mind as a key to diagnosing your bodily illness. Medical attitudes changed during the industrial revolution: mechanisation and scientific enquiry prompted a different idea of a healthy person. Humans were now likened to machines composed of separate working parts which sometimes malfunctioned. Treatment consisted of effecting repair to the damaged part, without considering the whole 'machine'. As the practice of *autopsy* developed, doctors began to associate specific diseases with particular organs or parts of the body, thereby building up the detailed knowledge which forms the basis of modern surgery.

Autopsy: a surgical examination of the body to establish the cause of death.

In the long history of health care, Western medicine, the type of medical practice most widely used in all industrialised countries, is a fairly recent development arising from the scientific thinking of the 17th and 18th centuries. Indeed, the reliance on curative drugs that we now associate with modern medicine dates from the early 20th century, with the discovery of germ-killing chemicals and the birth of the pharmaceutical industry. Traditional medicine has a history of several thousand years, with roots in the ancient civilisations of China, India, Egypt and Greece. Although lacking in the precise scientific understanding of disease, traditional medicine employed a wide range of techniques, some of which were clearly ineffective or even harmful whilst others contained insights into the workings of the human mind and body which still baffle modern science. The traditional practices of acupuncture, healing and herbal medicine are enjoying a resurgence of interest in the industrialised world, alongside more recent *alternative therapies* such as homoeopathy, osteopathy and psychotherapy. In the late 20th century, Western medicine is undergoing a period of change in which the value of traditional treatments is being rediscovered and new, holistic therapies – recognising the intimate connection between mind and body – are being tried.

Throughout the developing world, traditional medicine has been, for centuries, the mainstay of health care and is still widely and successfully practised. The 'barefoot doctors' in China readily combine acupuncture and herbal remedies with treatment by Western drugs. Since independence in Zimbabwe, traditional healers – discredited as 'witch doctors' by previous colonial governments – have been incorporated into the national health service. In India and Sri Lanka there are as many qualified practitioners of *Ayurveda*, a medical system developed over three thousand years ago, as there are doctors trained in Western methods. *Ayurveda*, meaning 'the science of life', takes into account each patient's physical, emotional and spiritual make-up when prescribing medicines derived from certain plants and spices. So ten patients suffering from the same symptoms may be treated with ten different remedies; the treatment, as in much traditional and alternative medicine, is geared to the patient, not the disease.

Traditional medicine is particularly valuable in the developing world because it is based on products that are cheap and available locally, it employs the accepted wisdom of generations and is generally free from side effects. But Western scientific research is also discovering that traditional plant-based remedies contain substances

Some common plants on which medicine depends for present and future drugs. The seeds of the cotton plant could provide a new male contraceptive.

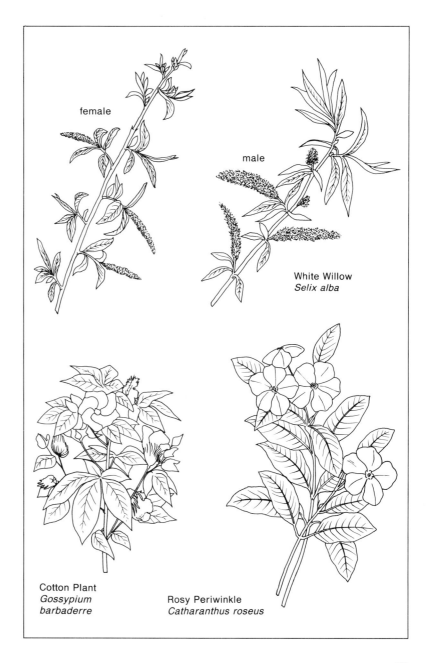

female

male

White Willow
Selix alba

Cotton Plant
Gossypium barbaderre

Rosy Periwinkle
Catharanthus roseus

which are of considerable value in treating the diseases of the industrialised world. Research into traditional plant drugs is increasing, particularly in the species-rich tropical rainforest, in the hope that a natural product will reveal a previously unknown chemical compound that will form the basis of a new treatment for heart disease, cancer or AIDS. The clinically packaged pills and bottled liquids seem worlds apart from the steamy rainforest, yet about 30% of modern medicines are based on plant products while more than 80% were originally derived from plants. It is to plants – and to traditional plant knowledge – that Western medicine is indebted for products such as pain-killers, anti-cancer drugs and the contraceptive pill. The active ingredient in aspirin was first isolated from the bark of the White Willow tree; successful treatment of two types of cancer, Hodgkin's disease and leukaemia, is based on an alkaloid found in the small flowering plant Rosy Periwinkle; and birth control was revolutionised by the discovery of diosgenin, the basis of the contraceptive pill, in the Mexican yam. Compared with the plant knowledge of traditional healers, however, Western understanding is still in its infancy.

Alternative medicine

As a reaction to the prevailing *mechanistic* view of human health – seeing the body as a machine whose damaged parts can be repaired by drugs or surgery – alternative medicine has flourished in the last quarter of the 20th century. Under the banner of alternative therapies comes a diverse group of treatments, some employing the wisdom of traditional practices, others using insights from more recent understanding of the human psyche. Common to most

I've called this emergency meeting, ladies and gentlemen, because of a serious outbreak of alternative medicine in this area.

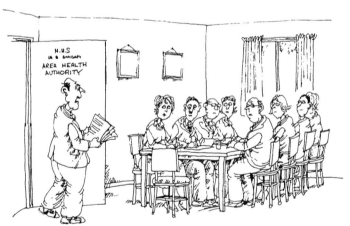

alternative techniques, though, is a holistic approach which regards the human being as a *system* rather than a machine. All parts of the system, according to this way of thinking, are constantly interacting and affecting each other; a physical problem, therefore, also affects the mind, and vice versa. It is no good, the argument continues, simply treating the *symptom* of disease; cancer cells may be attacked by specific drugs or radiation, but the likelihood of their recurrence is high unless the underlying causes – environmental, emotional and biological – are also addressed. Treatment, therefore, has to consider patients' psychological make-up, their lifestyle and diet, their personal relationships and their past history.

Homoeopathy

Developed by a German doctor, Samuel Hahnemann, in the late 18th century, homoeopathy works on the principle of 'treating like with like'. A homoeopathic remedy produces the same symptoms as those the sick person complains of, thereby provoking the body into shaking them off. Remedies are made from natural substances (some 3000 in all) which are diluted many hundreds of times, the greater the dilution the more potent the remedy is thought to be. Homoeopathic medicines are free from side effects and can therefore be bought without prescription; the right medicine, however, depends upon a patient's physical and emotional make-up as well as the symptoms of disease. Homoeopathy can treat a wide range of physical and mental conditions and is widely used in many European countries, India, South Africa and South America.

Herbal medicine

Remedies prepared from plant extracts form the basis of traditional medicine throughout the world. Animals, too, seek out the curative properties of certain plants. Homoeopathy uses an extensive range of plants; some are still used in the manufacture of Western drugs. Herbal medicine is an ancient practice which can be beneficial both for specific complaints and for general health. Some remedies are commonplace, such as mint for indigestion, sage for sore throats, garlic for coughs and colds; others require a concoction of many plants. Nicholas Culpeper, a 17th-century astrologer and London doctor, wrote an authoritative guide to herbal remedies, still in use today. Other therapies using herbal extracts are *aromatherapy*, which utilises the sense of smell as a healing force, and the *Bach flower remedies* – a collection of 38 remedies discovered by Dr Edward Bach which use the healing energy within certain flowers to treat personality disorders.

Acupuncture, acupressure

Acupuncture has been used in China for some 6000 years. Central to this therapy is the belief that the energy of life (*chi'i*) flows throughout the body along pathways, or meridians. When the meridians become blocked, illness occurs. The energy flow can be released through the insertion of fine needles in some of the 600 acupuncture points sited all over the body. Acupuncture is particularly effective in treating conditions not related to a specific disease. Still widely practised in China, it is gaining in popularity in the West. Acupressure (also known by its Japanese name of *Shiatsu*) works on the same principle of energy flows, but instead of needles, finger pressure is used at the appropriate points. The healing power of touch is considered important, as it is in *reflexology*, a therapy based on the belief that the body's organs can be healed through stimulating points in the patient's feet.

Spiritual healing

One of the oldest forms of health treatment, spiritual healing (also called *'the laying-on of hands'*) involves the patient's life energy being directed by the healer's hands, which are placed on or just above the surface of the patient's body. Healers believe that the human body contains, and is surrounded by, an energy field (or aura) that bulges or breaks if a person is ill. In Aruvedic medicine (the traditional medicine of India) there are seven energy centres, known as *chakras*, which the healer uses to re-direct or complete the patient's energy flow. Spiritual healing has proven effective in treating chronically ill patients for whom Western medicine has failed. Although inexplicable in conventional scientific terms, the powers of the healer are now being recognised and used in some hospitals.

Osteopathy and chiropractice

These therapies involve manipulating the spine and other bones through a combination of forceful movement of joints and gentle massage of muscles and tissue. It is believed that a lot of physical problems, particularly backache, are caused by incorrect standing or sitting postures which are then aggravated by stress and tension. Osteopathy and chiropractice aim not only to rectify damaged bone and muscle structures but also to restore the body's harmony.

Visualisation and meditation

Treatments which are based upon the healing power of the patient's own mind use these techniques extensively. In visualisation, patients create mental pictures of their illness and suitable images of the disease being attacked or eradicated; meditation is a process of removing the distractions of everyday life so that the mind can focus completely on something, e.g. a healing image. Such techniques have been shown to result in physical improvements as well as mental and emotional calmness. Relaxation aids, such as yoga or music, are often incorporated.

Psychotherapy and counselling

These represent a range of 'talking therapies' that have been developed to treat mental and emotional illnesses without the use of drugs. The therapist encourages patients to talk about their problems and, through sensitive guidance and coaxing, to discover and work towards their own solutions. Sometimes the therapy takes place in groups or with whole families. Such treatments are being used more frequently to help people come to terms with traumatic experiences, such as accidents or bereavements. *Hypnotherapy* uses similar techniques, but the patient is first put into a state of hypnosis so that subconscious feelings and anxieties can be expressed.

In the Western medical profession the effectiveness of alternative therapies is a matter of considerable debate and disagreement. Because some, such as healing and homoeopathy, defy current scientific explanations, they are often dismissed as worthless. Others, such as the latest psychotherapy techniques, are too new to have received official medical approval. All these treatments have their devout disciples, people who can claim that their health has been dramatically improved – the 'miracle cures', so called because we do not understand how they have worked. Perhaps more significant than these one-off cases, however, is the growing number of people who are turning to alternative therapies either out of despair at the failure of Western medicine to solve their particular problem or through an interest in pursuing more holistic, less drug-dependent health care.

Naturopathy: helping yourself to good health

Although differing in their techniques, alternative therapies all share a belief in *naturopathic* medicine – assisting the body to heal itself – rather than the *allopathic* tradition of Western medicine, whereby drugs are administered to counteract the effects of a disease. Naturopathy is based on the view that disease is the outward symbol of a breakdown in the natural harmony of the healthy mind and body, the balance between *yin* and *yang* according to Chinese philosophy. Whereas an allopathic treatment attempts to 'conquer' disease by 'attacking' it with external agents (drugs, surgery), naturopathic techniques try to help patients use their own inner resources to restore harmony and balance. The treatment of cancer provides a good example of the two methods. Allopathic medicine bombards cancer cells with chemicals and radiation, or removes the cancerous growth altogether; the naturopathic way, pioneered by American cancer specialist Carl Simonton and psychotherapist Stephanie Simonton, is for patients to use relaxation and visualisation techniques to enable their own immune system to overcome the cancer cells. There are many recorded examples of the success of this approach, though many Western specialists remain sceptical.

In any naturopathic treatment the whole person is considered, not just the diseased organ. A patient's self-image and outlook on life is explored and attention given to their lifestyle, including balance between work and leisure, management of stress and diet. Healthy eating is regarded as an essential component of a naturopathic approach, as are aerobic exercise and physical and mental relaxation. Considerable responsibility is placed on patients to 'own' the disease – to accept that they are unwell, to try to understand the underlying causes and to work out and maintain an appropriate programme of healing. Compared with the allopathic approach, in which patients build up a psychological dependence on the doctor and the drugs to make them well, naturopathy shifts the onus of healing more towards the patient.

Complementary medicine: the best of both worlds?

Few people in the industrialised world rely solely on alternative medicine. To do so would be to deny the tremendous advances made by Western medicine in immunisation against infectious diseases and

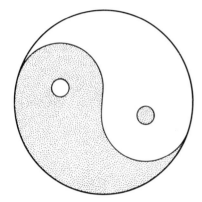

The yin-yang *symbol. According to ancient Chinese philosophy, all things are regulated by patterns of change.* Yin *and* yang *are the outer limits – once a process of change has reached* yin, *the direction of change swings back in favour of* yang. *In this way, change going too far in one direction is prevented and balance is maintained. The* yin-yang *idea has become influential in alternative health movements of the late 20th century.*

in the relief of suffering that modern drugs and surgery can achieve. There is a growing trend, however, towards incorporating the ideas and techniques of alternative medicine into Western medical practice, accepting that each has its strengths and weaknesses. This blend of the traditional and the modern, of Eastern and Western thinking, is called *complementary medicine*. In the treatment of cancer, patients are encouraged to use visualisation techniques in addition to receiving radiotherapy; spiritual healers are now working alongside specialists in some hospitals; a growing number of Western doctors are doing an additional training in homoeopathy; and psychotherapy techniques are used as an adjunct to drugs and electro-convulsive therapy (ECT) in treating the mentally ill.

Another facet of complementary medicine is the growth of interest in self-help techniques designed to enable people to live more healthily in polluted, stressful environments. Dietary plans, aerobics programmes, yoga and massage classes are all means by which ordinary people can assume more responsibility for their own health. In doing so they begin to view health holistically, though most would probably still seek Western medical expertise for a serious illness. Therein lies a problem for complementary medicine: the marrying of two different philosophies and often contradictory of health care. Is the naturopathic emphasis on diet, relaxation and visualisation of any real benefit to a patient whose immune system is then bombarded with alien chemicals? Alternative therapies have provided a timely challenge to Western medical thinking but it remains to be seen how well these two distinctive approaches can work together.

You look remarkably healthy, Mrs Brown – I hope you haven't been seeing another doctor?

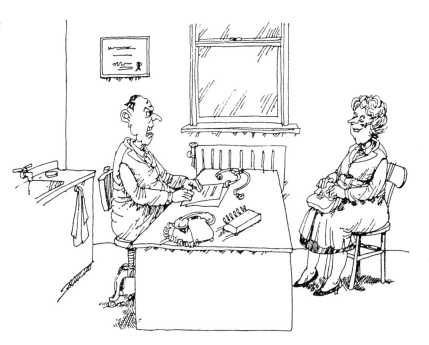

9 Health for all in the 21st century

The story so far

The evidence presented throughout this book clearly indicates that we are not going to achieve the WHO goal of 'health for all by the year 2000', set at the Thirtieth World Health Assembly in 1977. Perhaps it was always unrealistic, an over-ambitious target. Perhaps the goal was never meant to be *achieved*, but was set to serve as a rallying cry to inspire those responsible for health care around the world. Whatever the original intention, it is unlikely that any participant in that 1977 Assembly could have predicted the developments which have taken place since that date and whose impact has made the goal even more difficult to attain. Let us briefly review these unforeseen global trends and their impact on world health.

- *Poverty* remains the single most critical factor and since 1977 the gap between rich and poor has widened. Whilst GNP per capita grew, on average, by more than 2% per year in the industrialised

An impossible dream?

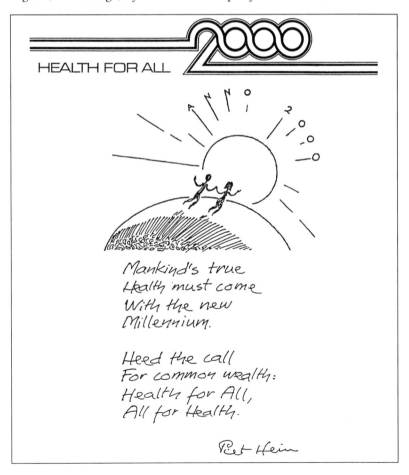

HEALTH FOR ALL 2000

Mankind's true Health must come with the new Millennium.

Heed the call for common wealth: Health for All, All for Health.

Piet Hein

nations during the 1980s, it declined annually in more than half of the developing countries over the same period. To make matters worse, the combination of high expenditure on defence and debt repayments is crippling their chances of economic recovery. Within wealthy countries, recent evidence points to an increase in the number of people living below the poverty line.

- *Basic needs* are still not being met. Despite sustained international campaigns, one-third of the world's people lack safe water and sanitation. An increase in public awareness about famine in Africa has not resulted in a decrease in the number of people whose lives are prematurely ended or devalued by prolonged malnutrition.

- *Urbanisation* has accelerated as the poor and unemployed flock to the major cities in search of a living. Urban growth is greatest in those cities, such as Mexico City, São Paulo and Calcutta, which are least able to provide for the newcomers' needs. Overcrowded shanty towns with few basic facilities are ripe for the spread of disease.

- *Education* suffered during the 1980s as a result of cuts in government expenditure, particularly in the poorer countries. More children now face the prospect of never acquiring the basic skills needed for their own and their societies' development. Some industrialised countries have reported a recent rise in the number of illiterate adults.

- *Environmental degradation* is not a new phenomenon, but its long-term harm to people and the planet has been only recently understood. Polluted environments are now known to be contributory factors in a wide range of degenerative diseases, particularly cancers.

- *New viruses*, such as the AIDS virus HIV, have emerged to baffle medical science and pose new threats to world health. Long-established diseases such as malaria continue to claim millions of lives due to the biological adaptability of the disease-carrying organisms.

Each of these trends is likely to have had a negative impact on health, but they do not exist separately; together, their cumulative effect has been disastrous. Undeniably, progress has been made towards the goal of 'health for all': immunisation and oral rehydration therapy programmes have saved millions of young lives; primary health care systems have given some of the poorest people access to medical care and knowledge; among the wealthier, greater personal responsibility for health is being exercised through attention to diet, fitness and lifestyle; and biotechnology continues to discover drugs and vaccines to prolong and improve the quality of our lives. However, this progress – mainly in the control and prevention of disease – is being undermined continually by the wider social and environmental trends outlined above. Every step forward is accompanied by at least half a pace backwards. To make faster progress, we need to have a broader understanding of what makes us, and our society, 'healthy'.

Healthy person, healthy planet

When we talk about 'health' we are usually referring to personal health, the physical and mental well-being of an individual. To understand a person's state of health, however, it seems evident that we need to look far beyond the individual, to appreciate the influences of immediate family and community, of society and of the planet as a whole. At all of these levels there are degrees of health and ill-health. A healthy family is not simply one in which individual members enjoy good physical and mental health but also one where loving and satisfying relationships, open communication and respect for each other's rights exist. A healthy society not only cares for the sick but also looks after those in poverty and ensures that education, housing and employment are equally available to all. A healthy planet, of course, is made up of healthy individuals, families and societies, all of whom demonstrate a respect for and cherish the natural resources and other life-forms which constitute Earth.

The significance of this holistic view of health is that all levels are *interrelated and interdependent*. As the diagram below illustrates, disease can occur at any level and its impact will be felt at all other levels. Ultimately, then, social and planetary disease *will directly impair the health of individuals*; likewise, unhealthy people will create unhealthy societies. This model of health helps to explain the disappointing rate of progress towards the goal of 'health for all by the year 2000', for it can be judged that insufficient emphasis has been placed on achieving health at the social and planetary levels. The model also provides a vision of 'health for all in the 21st

Factors influencing health at three levels.

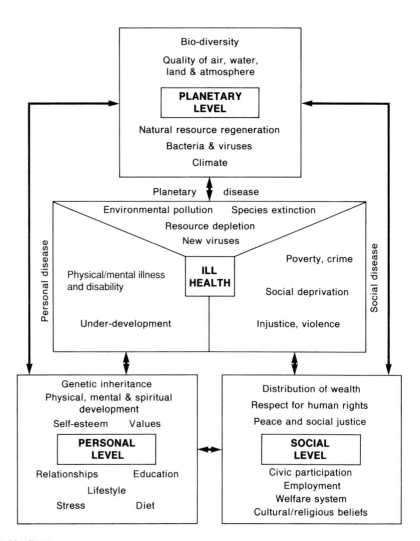

century', in which disease prevention and eradication should happen at all three levels at the same time. 'Health' might then be defined not in solely personal terms but as *a state of harmony between human beings, their societies and the environment*. This goes beyond the WHO definition of health as 'a state of complete physical, mental and social well-being' to incorporate the idea of people, communities and the environment all being part of one global system. The system is healthy when there is a state of harmony or balance between all parts of the system; when there is disharmony, there is *dis-ease*. It is interesting to note that the word 'health' originates from the Greek *holos*, meaning 'whole'. Perhaps the holistic vision of health described here gets closer to what the Greeks – the so-called 'fathers of modern medicine' – actually meant.

Towards the 'Healthy School'

A holistic definition of health can be applied to any social institution, from schools to industrial companies, from community organisations to governments. At a conference in Toronto in 1984 the idea of 'Healthy Cities' was first put forward. A Healthy City is defined as 'one that is continuously creating resources which enable people to support each other in performing all the functions of life and developing themselves to the maximum potential'. At a fundamental level a city is unhealthy if it cannot provide its citizens with the basic needs of personal health – safe water and sanitation, adequate food, shelter and sufficient employment. The Healthy City concept goes much further in suggesting that health is also dependent on a range of other social and environmental factors which affect the quality of people's lives. A recent national survey discovered what British city dwellers considered to be the most important characteristics. The results are shown in the tables below and on the following page.

Factors affecting the quality of life in British cities

Percentage of respondents rating dimensions as very important or important

Dimension	Very important	Important or very important
Violent crime	78.2	93.3
Health facilities	70.1	93.5
Non-violent crime	76.9	92.9
Pollution	55.3	88.8
Cost of living	54.8	87.3
Shopping facilities	49.4	86.7
Racial harmony	52.0	80.2
Scenic quality	39.2	78.2
Cost of owner-occupied housing	50.0	73.9
Wage levels	49.6	70.2
Education facilities	50.5	69.7
Employment prospects	52.6	69.2
Unemployment levels	44.2	67.0
Sports facilities	33.1	66.5
Leisure facilities	24.2	62.7
Travel-to-work time	37.7	62.4
Quality of council housing	29.3	53.0
Access to council housing	27.6	48.3
Cost of private rented accommodation	20.8	44.2

Rankings of British cities for quality of life

Using the dimensions in the first table, and the weighting given to each, this is how British cities would score for their 'quality of life'.

1	Edinburgh	14	Portsmouth	27	Leeds
2	Aberdeen	15	Southampton	28	Sunderland
3	Plymouth	16	Southend	29	Bolton
4	Cardiff	17	Hull	30	Manchester
5	Hamilton – Motherwell	18	Aldershot – Farnborough	31	Liverpool
6	Bradford	19	Bristol	32	Nottingham
7	Reading	20	Derby	33	Newcastle
8	Stoke-on-Trent	21	Norwich	34	London
9	Middlesborough	22	Birkenhead	35	Wolverhampton
10	Sheffield	23	Blackpool	36	Coventry
11	Oxford	24	Luton	37	Walsall
12	Leicester	25	Glasgow	38	Birmingham
13	Brighton	26	Bournemouth		

Source: Streetwise (Bulletin of the National Association for Urban Studies), no. 3, Summer 1990.

So what does the Healthy School look like? Below are ten suggested dimensions – you may want to add more of your own. You can then use this chart as a checklist, giving each dimension a score from 0 to 5 according to how well you think your school rates in carrying out these tasks. Compare your scores with those of your friends and teachers. Is your school healthy? If there is room for improvement – as there surely will be – what can *you* do and what needs to be done by others, including teachers, parents, community or council officials and the government? Are these improvements achievable and affordable and, if so, who should pay any costs incurred? Creating the Healthy School is not going to be easy, but simply working towards it will ensure better health for all.

The Healthy School is one which:

- enables all students to develop their full potential
- fosters co-operative and humane relationships amongst students and between teachers and students
- respects the rights of all members of the school community and expects them to fulfil their responsibilities
- promotes equal opportunities and disallows discrimination on the grounds of disability, gender, race or sexuality
- provides additional support for students with emotional, social or learning problems
- promotes healthy eating and healthy living
- provides sound guidance on all aspects of personal hygiene, disease prevention, social and sexual relationships
- encourages democratic participation by students in the running of the school
- provides a clean, comfortable and pleasing place to work
- is environmentally conscious in its use of energy and other resources.

Further resources on health issues

Introductory reading

AIDS and Development, CAFOD Information Pack, 1990. Well-presented information on AIDS in the developing world.

Behrman, N. *Health in Developing Countries... in Perspective*, Hobsons, 1988. Sound discussion of causes and impact of ill-health; good case studies and illustrations.

Children First!, UK Committee for Unicef. Free quarterly magazine containing some interesting articles on maternal and child health.

Discussion sheets on health and related issues are published by Christian Aid, Centre for World Development Education and Oxfam. Ideal for project work.

Fyson, N.L. *World Health and Population*, Batsford, 1986. Wide-ranging and informative, but uncritical, survey of health and population issues.

Hampton, J. *World Health*, Wayland World Issues, 1987. Covers the major issues in brief, easy-to-read style.

New Internationalist. Excellent monthly magazine on global issues with clearly presented arguments and facts. Health features prominently in many numbers.

World Health, WHO. Bi-monthly magazine with an emphasis on promoting preventive health care.

More advanced reading

AIDS and the Third World, Panos, 1988. Comprehensive global review, though statistics and forecasts inevitably out of date.

Chaitow, L. *Clear Body, Clear Mind*, Gaia, 1990. Informative self-help manual on keeping healthy in a polluted world.

Chetley, A. *A Healthy Business? World Health and the Pharmaceutical Industry*, Zed Books, 1990. Detailed and authoritative analysis of the global drugs trade.

Children and the Environment, UNEP/Unicef, 1990. Useful summaries and statistics on environment-related disease.

Garfield, R., and G. Williams, *Health and Revolution. The Nicaraguan Experience*, Oxfam, 1989. Interesting account of primary health care development against enormous odds.

Hammond, J., and L. Reveco (eds.), *Harsh Treatment. The Politics of Health*, Third World First, 1988. Short articles clearly showing the links between health, politics and power throughout the world.

Leshan, L. *Holistic Health. How to Understand and Use the Revolution in Medicine*, Turnstone, 1984. Interesting analysis of the limitations of conventional medicine.

Taylor, P. *The Smoke Ring. Tobacco, Money and Multinational Companies*, Sphere, 1985. Lively investigation of the struggle between health promotion and wealth creation.

Werner, D. *Where There is no Doctor*, Macmillan, 1980. The classic handbook for community health workers.

World Health Forum, WHO. Quarterly journal containing informative and readable articles written by health care experts.

Facts and figures

Health issues generate an abundance of facts and figures which can be overwhelming. In addition to the books and journals listed above, the following are reliable and user-friendly sources.

Balding, J. *Young People in 1990*, HEA Schools Health Education Unit, University of Exeter. Annual report of survey of 'health related behaviour' conducted amongst 11–16 year olds.

Health Education Authority leaflets and pamphlets on significant health matters for young people in the UK. Good sources of basic information.

The State of the World's Children 1992, Unicef/Oxford University Press. Annual report with excellent case studies and statistical tables on child and maternal health.

Simulation game

Juvenis – the Wonder Drug, Centre for Global Education, 1987. Explores the dubious ethics and politics surrounding the introduction of a fictitious anti-ageing drug.

Software

Malaria, Centre for World Development Education. An interactive programme exploring the factors behind the transmission of malaria. BBC version only.

World Development Database, Centre for World Development Education. Statistics on 16 social and economic indicators for 129 countries. A3000 and Nimbus versions.

Films and videos

Concord Video and Film Council has an extensive range of films and videos on health issues for sale or hire. The following list is a selection.

AIDS – an African Perspective, video, 52 minutes, 1988. How attitudes to sex help spread the disease, and what governments are doing to fight it.

Alternatives – Holistic Healing, video, 30 minutes, 1984. Part of a series, this video introduces many alternative therapies.

Bitter Harvest – Pesticides and the Third World, video, 22 minutes, 1987. Comprising slides which indicate the need to control the export and use of dangerous pesticides.

Cancer Prevention Clinic, video, 26 minutes, 1984. Features the work of a British clinic whose leader argues that cancer results from unhealthy lifestyles.

For Export Only – Pills, film/video, 55 minutes, 1981. How drug companies sell to the developing world products that are banned elsewhere.

Nicaragua – the Other Invasion, video, 33 minutes, 1984. Looks at the tragic impact of the Contras' war on real progress in primary health care.

Picture of Health, video, 50 minutes each part. An 8-part series arguing that the treatment of ill-health, in both rich and poor countries, needs social and political action as well as medical care for the individual.

Primary Health Care – a Team Approach, film/video, 38 minutes, 1983. Features the community health care programme conducted by a London health centre.

Smoking – a Double Standard, film/video, 30 minutes. The marketing of cigarettes by British-American tobacco companies in the developing world.

To Taste a Hundred Herbs – Gods, Ancestors and Medicine in a Chinese Village, video, 58 minutes, 1986. Focuses on the village doctor who integrates traditional Chinese and Western medicine in his successful treatments.

Organisations

The following organisations provide information and resources (many mentioned in this section) on health care and health issues. When writing, be as specific as possible in your request.

Action on Disability and Development (ADD), 23 Lower Keyford, Frome, Somerset BA11 4AP.

Action on Smoking and Health (ASH), 5–11 Mortimer Street, London W1N 7RN.

Baby Milk Action (BMAC), 6 Regent Terrace, Cambridge CB2 1AA.

Catholic Fund for Overseas Development (CAFOD), 2 Romero Close, Stockwell Road, London SW9 9TY.

Centre for Global Education (CGE), University of York, Heslington, York YO1 5DD.

Centre for World Development Education (CWDE), 1 Catton Street, London WC1R 4AB.

Christian Aid, PO Box 100, London SE1 7RT.

Concord Video and Film Council, 201 Felixstowe Road, Ipswich IP3 9BJ.

Health Education Authority (HEA), Hamilton House, Mabledon Place, London WC1H 9TX.

HEA Schools Health Education Unit, School of Education, University of Exeter, Heavitree Road, Exeter EX1 2LU.

Life Education Centres, PO Box 137, London N10 3JJ. (Preventive drug abuse programmes.)

New Internationalist Publications, 120–126 Lavender Avenue, Mitcham, Surrey CR4 3HP.

Oxfam, 274 Banbury Road, Oxford OX2 7DZ.

Terrence Higgins Trust, 52–54 Gray's Inn Road, London WC1X 8JU. (Information on AIDS.)

Third World First, 232 Cowley Road, Oxford OX4 1UH.

UK Committee for Unicef, 55–56 Lincoln's Inn Fields, London WC2A 3NB.

WaterAid, 1 Queen Anne's Gate, London SW1H 9BT.

World Health Organisation (WHO), Distribution and Sales, 1211 Geneva 27, Switzerland.

Index

acupuncture, 69
affluence, diseases of, 18–20, 23
AIDS, 7, 12, 31–9
allopathic medicine, 70
Alma-Ata Declaration, 58
alternative medicine, 68–71
alternative therapies, 66, 68–70
Anderton, James, 35
Ankrah, Dr Maxine, 39
antibiotics, 13, 15, 16, 56
Ayurveda, 66–7, 69
AZT, 39

baby milk, 56–7
'barefoot' doctors, 58, 66
Barnard, Dr Christiaan, 53
Bhopal accident, 47
biotechnology, 53

cancer, 12, 18–19, 20, 40, 45, 47–8, 53
    breast, 19, 20
    lung, 18–19, 20, 24, 25, 26, 47
    skin, 46, 47
    treatment of, 68, 70, 71
carcinogens, 48
Chernobyl accident, 47–8
CHILD-to-child programme, 60–1
childhood diseases, 6, 13, 15–16
chiropractice, 69
cholera, 43–4, 46
cigarette advertising, 24, 29–30
community health workers, 16, 58,
    59–61, 65
complementary medicine, 70–1
contraception, 12, 36–8, 62, 68
counselling, 69
curative medicine, 40, 52–3, 65

debt, 51, 63, 73
deficiency diseases, 16–17
degenerative diseases, 6, 11, 20, 40
development aid, 50–1, 52
diarrhoea, 15, 33, 44
drug companies, 11, 56–7
drugs, 24, 25, 26

education, 37, 62–4, 73
    of girls, 62–3, 64
elderly people, 11
electro-convulsive therapy (ECT), 21, 71
environment, 11, 19, 25, 40–9, 73
epidemics, 33

Facts for Life, 64

genital mutilation, 61

global warming, 46
Gulf War, 48

health
    definitions of, 5, 75
    expenditure on, 10, 21, 23, 29, 50–1,
        65
Healthy City, 75–6
Healthy School, 75–6
heart disease, 12, 18, 20, 24
herbal medicine, 69
HIV, 31, 32, 36, 38
holistic health, 9, 21, 66, 68, 70, 71,
    74–5
homelessness, 10
homoeopathy, 69, 71

immunisation, 7, 13, 15, 16
infant mortality, 7, 19
infant mortality rate, 18, 35, 62, 64–5
infectious diseases, 6, 13, 20
International Drinking Water Supply and
    Sanitation Decade, 9, 42–3

Johnson, Earvin ('Magic'), 36

Kenyan Water for Health Organisation, 42

leukaemia, 48, 68
life expectancy, 6, 7, 35, 65
literacy, 10, 12, 63, 64

Mahler, Dr Halfdan, 28, 52, 59, 65
malaria, 17, 33, 43, 46, 49
malnutrition, 16, 73
maternal mortality, 61
measles, 13, 14, 15, 18, 52
meditation, 69
melanoma, *see* cancer, skin
mental health, 10
mental illness and disability, 20–1
Morley, Dr David 52, 60

naturopathic medicine, 70
neuroses, 21
Nicot, Jean, 27
nicotine, 24
nutrition, 9, 13, 16

oral rehydration therapy (ORT), 15
organ transplants, 53–4
osteopathy, 69
ozone depletion, 46

parasitic diseases, 17–18
passive smoking, 25

pesticides, 43, 47, 48–9
plant-based medicines, 67–8, 69
polio, 7, 13, 14
pollution, 40
    of air, 44–6
    by cars, 45–6
    of water, 9, 17, 41–4
population, 8, 11
poverty, 15, 19, 62, 72
    diseases of, 15–19, 39
preventive medicine, 40, 52–3, 54, 59, 65
primary health care, 58–9, 61–2, 64–5
psychoses, 21
psychotherapy, 69, 71

quality of life, 54–5

racism, 21
respiratory infections, 16, 44, 45
rights, 25, 36, 61–2

Safe Motherhood Initiative, 61
sanitation, 9, 17, 40, 42–3, 73
self-help, 12, 71
sexual practices, 32, 34, 36, 37, 38, 62
Simonton, Carl and Stephanie, 70
smallpox, 7, 18, 33, 53
smoking, 20, 24–30
    and girls/women, 26
    and young people, 25, 26–7
social justice, 21, 59, 65
spiritual healing, 69

technology, 23, 52–4, 59, 65
tobacco companies, 27–8, 29–30
toxic waste, 44, 45, 47–9
traditional medicine, 66–8
tuberculosis (TB), 7, 13, 16, 18, 19

undernutrition, 16
urbanisation, 10, 73

viruses, 31, 40, 73
visualisation, 69, 71

water, 9, 17, 40, 41–4, 73
water-related disease, 15, 41, 42, 43
Western medicine, 66–8, 70, 71
Wilson, Michael, 54
women, 26, 38, 41, 42, 56–7, 61–2
World Conference on Education for All, 64
World Health Organisation (WHO), 5, 15,
    20–1, 28, 30, 72
World Summit for Children, 22

yin and yang, 70